The Visual Cortices

The Visual Cortices

Edison K. Miyawaki, M.D.

Copyright © 2020 by Edison K. Miyawaki, M.D.

Library of Congress Control Number:		2020900433
ISBN:	Hardcover	978-1-7960-8175-6
	Softcover	978-1-7960-8176-3
	eBook	978-1-7960-8181-7

All rights reserved. No part of this book may be reproduced or transmitted in any form or by any means, electronic or mechanical, including photocopying, recording, or by any information storage and retrieval system, without permission in writing from the copyright owner.

The views expressed in this work are solely those of the author and do not necessarily reflect the views of the publisher, and the publisher hereby disclaims any responsibility for them.

Any people depicted in stock imagery provided by Getty Images are models, and such images are being used for illustrative purposes only.
Certain stock imagery © Getty Images.

Print information available on the last page.

Rev. date: 01/15/2020

To order additional copies of this book, contact:
Xlibris
1-888-795-4274
www.Xlibris.com
Orders@Xlibris.com

CONTENTS

1. Parieto-Occipital and Calcarine Sulci 1
2. The Limits of Gennari's Stripe 6
3. Meridians 9
4. Elementary Clarification 15
5. The Origin of Streams 18
6. A Note on Geniculocalcarine and Corticogeniculate 24
7. A Task 26
8. Distinguishing Features of an Area 32
9. Omission Correction 39
10. Why WHAT and WHERE? 45
11. Two Problems with Diagrams 52
12. The Many Disorders of Higher Visual Processing 57

References 65

1

Parieto-Occipital and Calcarine Sulci

This monograph is the fifth in a series. The idea of the series as a whole is to think about human neuroanatomy uniquely, at times along the lines of traditional textbooks, but not always.

*

If I say, in the off-the-rack manner that was my style for too long, that a first task in evaluating a visual problem is to localize a lesion either anterior or posterior to the optic chiasm (or at the optic chiasm), a critic couldn't object that I'm wrong. Yet by saying so, I don't reach into a data trove which, over the last century in particular, has accrued to the point that we now have a better idea than ever before about how the cerebral cortex works *anatomically*[1]–and not just in terms of vision.

---

1 Maybe the adverb is wrong: anatomy is anatomy; anatomy doesn't "work," one could argue.
A colleague has opined that "[c]ortical physiologists often claim—whether or not it is true—that in studying a particular area they hope to discover general principles of cortical function" (Born and Bradley, 2005; the first author works at the school next to my hospital). To hope one discovers general principles isn't to succeed in doing so, alas. Nevertheless, there are anatomical aspects of the visual cortices that show up elsewhere in non-visual cortex. Maybe there are organizational principles that contribute to how the cortex does, in fact, *work*.

(There's a relationship, not an either/or choice, between what happens anteriorly and posteriorly in the quite connected visual pathway.)

In what follows, we'll discuss visual neuroanatomy in humans, with a focus on cortex or, more accurately, the *cortices* in the vicinity of the **parieto-occipital sulcus (or fissure)**, the latter best visualized when looking medially at a human hemibrain.

Let's locate the fissure in a midsagittal section chosen to exaggerate our structure of interest:

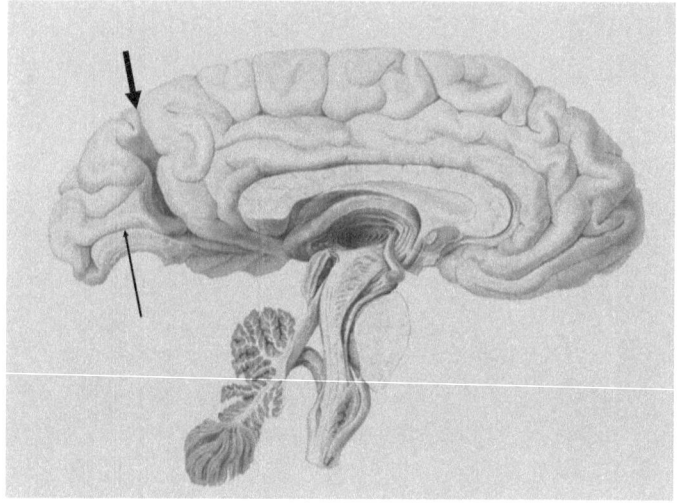

The thicker arrow indicates the superior extent of parieto-occipital sulcus.

Where would you say that **calcarine sulcus** begins and ends?

Part of it, but not the start of it, is marked by the thin, longer arrow.

My question has to do with the relationship between calcarine sulcus and **striate cortex**–"striate," because **stripes (or lines) of Gennari** lie along both superior/dorsal and inferior/ventral cortical banks of the "**body**" of calcarine sulcus (the longer, thinner arrow points to that "body"). Looking specifically at Gennari's own image, published in 1784, where is his line ("F" refers to white matter)? In the right image (a copy of the left one), the arrowhead sits on a white line of Gennari—subtle, wouldn't you say?

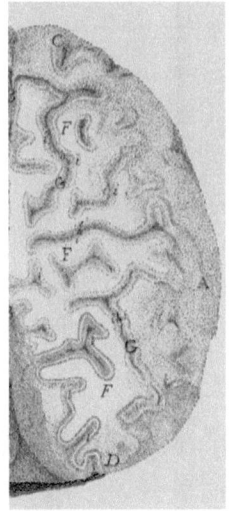 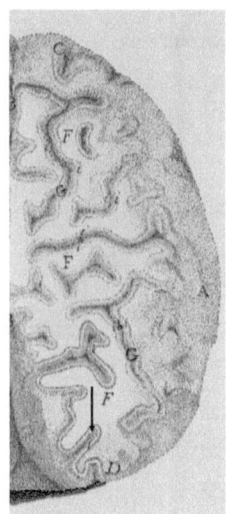

Here's another way of asking the same thing: where does **primary visual cortex** (primary visual cortex is also known as striate cortex; it's *also* known as **Brodmann's area number 17**, or **V1**); . . . where does primary-visual-striate cortex, Brodmann's area 17, viz., V1, begin and end?[2]

*

Some history helps us:

> In the classical anatomical studies conducted at the beginning of the Twentieth Century, the relation of the calcarine sulcus to the striate cortex was the subject of intense investigation. These studies showed that

---

2 And if there's a V1, there must be others like 2, 3, 4, 5, or more, right? Keep reading. I'm interested in NOT generating a stock image, which a person can find in any Google search, of where all the visual cortices supposedly are located in humans. I'd emphasize "supposedly are," because how does one know for a fact where they are located?

the anterior calcarine sulcus, i.e., the extension of the calcarine sulcus anterior to the point of intersection with the parieto-occipital fissure, is the border between limbic cortex lying on the isthmus and the striate cortex, which is found only on the ventral bank of the calcarine sulcus at this point. Caudal to the point of convergence of the parieto-occipital fissure with the calcarine sulcus, i.e., on the body of the calcarine sulcus, the striate cortex extends on both banks of the sulcus. The striate cortex extends outside the calcarine sulcus father caudally, i.e., close to the occipital pole (Iaria and Petrides, 2007).

The *anterior* **calcarine sulcus**? Where's that? And the **isthmus** of what? Paul Broca, no slouch of an anatomist, was aware of the anterior extent of a "scissure calcarine," marked as "K."

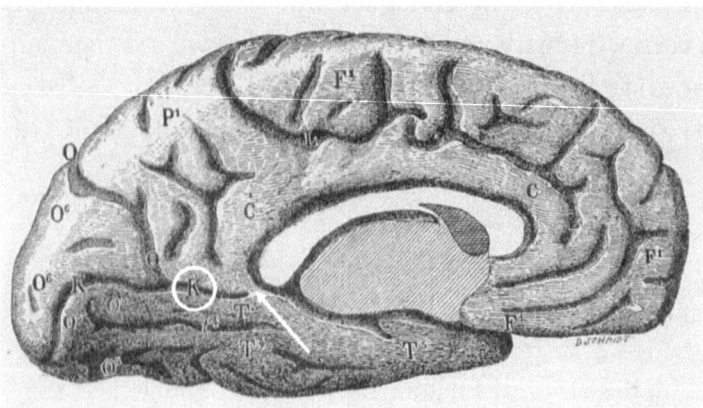

The arrow marks an isthmus of cingulate gyrus at the transition to **parahippocampal gyrus.**

Iaria and Patrides (2007) are interestingly precise: a stripe of Gennari is present only on the ventral cortical back of the *anterior* sulcus. In the body of calcarine sulcus, stripes can be seen in both its dorsal and ventral banks.

The Visual Cortices

*

A preoccupation over what's striate and what's not and where striate cortex is in relation to calcarine sulcus is hardly new, as Brodmann attests early in the early 20th century:

> Whereas in man [the striate area] is almost entirely limited to the medial side, and especially to the cortex of the calcarine sulcus, in monkeys (except the marmoset), and particularly in the great apes, by far its largest extent is on the lateral convexity, and it is divided approximately equally between medial and lateral surfaces in marmosets, lemurs and macrochiropterans [viz., most bats]. In carnivores the medial portion of the area is usually larger than the lateral (to a notable degree in the dog), as in man, and this is also the case in many ungulates [animals with hooves] (Brodmann, 2006, specifically p. 187).

By starting with a look at the human medial brain, we've already intimated that if you want to visualize human V1, it's best to think about it as an identifiable structure on the medial surface in parasagittal or midsagittal section. If you gaze at the posterior, medial surface of any human hemibrain, you'll discover:

calcarine sulcus, which anatomically relates to . . .

parieto-occipital sulcus or fissure;

and, in terms of V1 specifically, you see . . .

the stripes or lines of Gennari.

We've identified the first of the visual cortices.

2

The Limits of Gennari's Stripe

We only discuss striate cortex, just V1, which has its *largest* extent on the *lateral* convexity in some, but not all, monkeys and apes. Brodmann knew as much in 1909, as we learned in the first chapter. He also says (still on his p. 187) that, particularly in humans, striate cortex is "a field stuck on the occipital pole like a cap"—as it were, like the cap display at the end of an aisle in some store.

If V1 is present on the lateral convexity without question in many animals, then it's time to steal a metaphor from Tootell et al. (1996) regarding humans: if V1 were considered as a bed sheet, a noticeable difference in humans is that the V1 sheet has been pulled around either occipital pole, and has been tucked into the depths of medial calcarine sulcus on either side.

The main question/point is: what's anterior to—what's *around* V1 on *either* on the lateral or medial surfaces? Furthermore, can we reliably delineate borders between V1 and other visual cortices?

*

Is it imperfect to rely just on Gennari's stripe to indicate the extent of V1 in either monkey or human brain?

The rhetorically leading question has a stock answer:

> The current identifications of homologues in the human occipital cortex of the visual areas established in the monkey should be treated with caution and should be regarded as tentative suggestions, because the methodologies used in studies with monkeys and humans are very different. In the monkey, the definition of a cortical visual area is based on mapping of the visual field representation at the single-neuron level with microelectrode recording. In the human brain, attempts to map these same areas are usually based on global signal changes in fMRI, i.e., indirect measures of functional activity based on blood flow, and the precise location of an area is likely to be affected by the details of blood vessel distribution (Iaria and Petrides, 2007).

The authors say that identification of V1 depends on your method of seeing it.

Functional MRI aids visualization (e.g., Tootell et al., 1996, Coggan et al., 2017), but there are other methods. There's tracing of degenerated axons from unilateral occipital infarctions to discover a representation of the vertical meridian–a V1 border–in the undamaged, contralateral hemisphere (Clarke and Miklossy, 1990). There's post-mortem receptor mapping of human occipital cortex that examines uniquely V1 receptor profiles (e.g., Eickhoff et al., 2008). Of late, novel genetic delivery systems allow injection of a neuron, then the ability to trace its axonal or dendritic course, synapse by synapse, in either retrograde or anterograde direction (Nassi et al., 2015). Anatomists have long known that V1 on one side interlinks with ipsilateral/homolateral **lateral geniculate nucleus** of thalamus, but maybe V1 neurons have no less important connections to other areas of cortex.

*

What's around V1 has to do with what we can accurately identify as its border.

We'll be prudent *not* to oversimplify by saying that Brodmann's areas 18 and 19 lie sequentially anterior to area 17, although you could pull any neuroanatomy textbook off your shelf to find an image of Brodmann's areas 18 and 19 concentrically present around area 17 at the occipital pole.

3

Meridians

One couldn't indict Kaas (1996) for not speaking his mind. The numeration is his, not mine:

1. Early proposals on how extrastriate cortex [viz., that which is not striate cortex] is subdivided were inconsistent with each other, and differences in interpretation were not resolved.
2. Brodmann's proposal of two ring-like areas, 18 and 19, surrounding primary visual cortex gained great acceptance despite the lack of agreement among different investigators considering the same evidence.
3. The concepts of areas 18 and 19, transposed to signify V2 and V3, have had great impact on recent and even current theories of extrastriate visual cortex organization in primates.
4. Nevertheless, Brodmann's areas 18 and 19, as defined in humans and Old World monkeys [e.g., macaques], correspond to none of the fields currently proposed for these primates.
5. . . . we should recognize that V2 is about half the size of Brodmann's area 18 in Old World monkeys and humans.
6. Current concepts of V3 differ greatly from the ring-like area 19 of Brodmann. We question the validity and usefulness of retaining the concept of V3 in primates. . . ..

There is no point seven.

*

Evidence to justify a broadside against Brodmann's visual areas 17, 18, and 19 took years to collect, Kaas says. Peeking into that history, just for our purpose of delineating V1 from extrastriate or, as they otherwise called, "**prestriate**" cortices, we read about work dating to the 1960's (e.g., Myers, 1962 and Choudhury et al., 1965):

> Only the parts of area 17 very close to the border between areas 17 and 18 sent axons across to the other side [via corpus callosum], and these seemed to end, for the most part, in area 18, close to its border with area 17. If we assume that the input the cortex gets from the geniculates is strictly from contralateral visual fields–left field to right cortex and right field to left cortex–the presence of corpus-callosum connections between hemispheres should result in one hemisphere's receiving input from more than one-half the visual fields; the connections should produce an overlap in visual-field territories feeding into the two hemispheres. That is, in fact, what we find. Two electrodes, one in each hemisphere near the 17-18 borders, frequently record cells whose fields overlap by several degrees (Hubel, 1995).

Pause.

Brodmann based his famous Brodmann areas on differences in cytoarchitecture across the cortical mantle. The above excerpt doesn't talk at all about layering or other histo-architectural aspects. Instead, the take-home is that if you really want to discern the end of area 17 and the beginning of area 18 in, say, *right* occipital lobe, look where to both visual hemifields (both left *and* right visual hemifields) are represented in cortex, specifically at the border between right area 17 and 18. (The borderzone is technically in area 18.) The corpus callosum doesn't connect all areas of one area 17 to its contralateral cortical counterpart, because, frankly, what would be the use of that? Just the vertical midline between the two visual hemifields is represented at the border between areas 17 and 18.

But if cytoarchitecture isn't the be-all-end-all discrimination, what really is "an area"?

> There are at least five criteria which can be used to define a visual area. All these criteria can be applied to the striate cortex. They are (1) a well defined cytoarchitecture; (2) a complete map of the visual field; (3) a well defined anatomical input (in the case of the striate cortex an exclusive input from the lateral geniculate nucleus); (4) distinct functional properties and (5) callosal connections (Zeki, 1978).

The author goes on to lament that the five criteria, though met in the case of striate or V1 cortex, don't necessarily help define other areas, including Brodmann's areas 18 and 19. So, Kass, whom we quoted at the start of this chapter, doesn't sound quite so curmudgeonly as first seemed. No less than Zeki pronouncing his five criteria, Kass votes for as much clarity as possible without the possibility of being mislead by just one criterion.

*

Textbooks, on the other hand, attempt definitiveness, as in this example:

> ... the vertical meridian forms the border between the representations of the visual field in V1 and V2. The horizontal meridian separates areas V2 and V3. V2 and V3, like V1, consist of ventral and dorsal portions, which contain paired representations of the contralateral upper and lower quadrants. ... [S]ome of the borders of visual areas also could be established in the human brain by tracing callosal afferents from large lesions of the opposite occipital cortex. This is possible because the termination

of callosal fibres in V1-V4 shows a strong preference for the representations of the vertical meridian, i.e., for the V1/V2 and the outer V3 borders (Nieuwenhuys et al., 2008).

I know that we haven't discussed either V2 or V3 or the anatomical contiguity of V1, V2, and V3. We'll get to all that in chapter seven.

For now, consider what the textbook teaches. The representation of the vertical meridian in a view of the world in front of us . . .

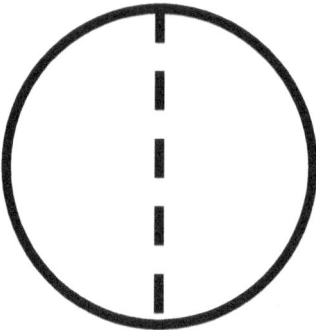

. . . isn't quite complete. We should include a horizontal meridian. The vertical meridian then divides into an upper part (black dashes) and a lower one (grey dashes):

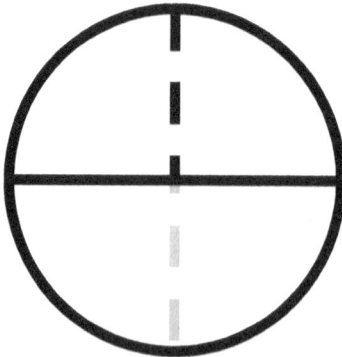

We know from basic neuroanatomy that upper visual space is represented in V1 below the calcarine sulcus and that lower visual space is represented in V1 above the calcarine sulcus. The vertical meridian at the border between V1 and V2 is likewise divided. Here's a schematized view; the medial occipital cortex is rendered as a box divided in half along its length by the calcarine sulcus (indicated by the thin line):

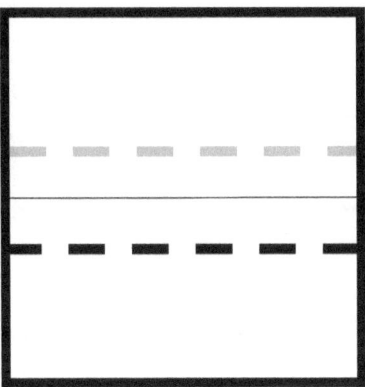

The textbook adds that representations of the vertical meridian *repeat* elsewhere in the occipital cortex. We'll add one iteration:

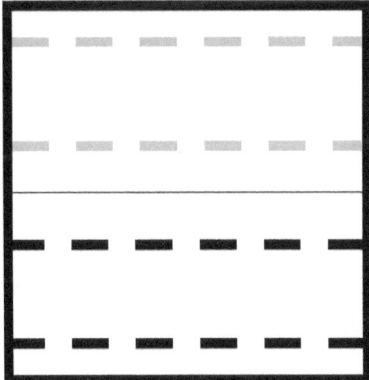

The horizontal meridian still matters. In fact, it's represented at the border between V2 and V3 (thin lines):

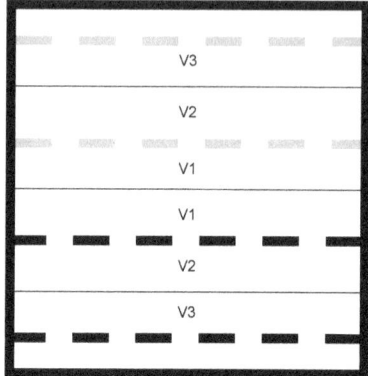

And, in human V1, representation of the horizontal meridian locates to the bottom of the calcarine sulcus.

Why there are multiple retinotopic representations is anyone's guess, but re-representation of sensory surfaces happens in mammalian neocortex generally (Allman and Kass, 1974).[3]

---

3 An obvious example of non-visual sensory re-representation would be Brodmann's areas 3a, 3b ("S1"), 1, and 2–all posterior to the central sulcus (discussed in Van Essen and Glasser, 2018).

4

Elementary Clarification

When experts talk about "'pre'-striate" they mean extrastriate. And by "pre"- or "extra"-striate, they don't refer to the route or routes via retina, optic nerve, optic tract, etc. to primary visual cortex, V1.

But we ended the last chapter referring to redundant visuotopic–which is to say, retinotopic–representations.[4] Let's put aside subtleties which we've mentioned–how the horizontal visual-field meridian separates V2 and V3, whereas representation of the vertical meridian marks the border between cortical areas V1 and V2. If you are quite eager, you can fast forward to chapter eight, where we address meridians again. If you would, though, read from start to finish: I'm trying to follow a reasonable line of thought.

If visuotopy/retinotopy happens over and over, then it shouldn't surprise that what happens in V1 and downstream from it has to do with what the retina allows us–or, in one instance in particular–*doesn't* allow us to visualize.

*

---

4   From Van Essen and Glasser (2018): "'Retinotopic' and 'visuotopic' are largely synonymous, and both terms are widely used. Retinotopic is appropriate when the mapping method involves visual stimulation via the retina. Visuotopic is more appropriate when the analysis involves connections or interactions between topographically organized visual areas, but without overt retinal stimulation."

It's the kind of experiment any grade schooler could perform; the earliest description that I've found dates to the 17th century:

1   0

Put your face at a comfortable distance from the page (about arm's length) as you gaze at the "1" and the "0" with both eyes open. Now close the left eye, but focus the right eye on the "1." Now move your face towards the page with the left eye still closed, and watch the "0" disappear. Yes, it's a demonstration of the blind spot in the right eye.

Edmund Mariotte's original description mandates that the right eye must remain "fixed and very steady" (a version of his report in English is Justin, 1668). In a 17th-century peer review, a certain Pecquet commented, "Every one wonders that no person before you has been aware of this privation of sight, which every one finds, now you have given notice of it." But, ever the reviewer, Pecquet objected to Mariotte's stated concern, that "there appears no reason to me why there should be no vision in the place of the optic nerve where it is . . .." Pecquet doesn't discuss the blind spot, which, we now know, is that place where there are no receptors to light, specifically at the optic disc. On the other hand, Mariotte does discuss the blind spot without quite realizing its significance: his experiment demonstrates that there is no vision in the place of the optic nerve head precisely where it is in the eye, but he wondered, moreover, whether vision happens in the retina at all. Pecquet opined that of course vision is retinal.

The "privation" in the experiment can be reversed in at least two ways. You could move your face away from the page (left eye still closed) thereby allowing a wider field of view. Or, as happens almost involuntarily, you might saccade the eyes even just for a moment to the "0," although the left eye is shut. Either way, privation reverses; "0" returns to view.

We can describe both phenomena in neuro-opthalmologic terms. If I move my head away, I perform the *opposite* of a *con*vergence. My eyes subtly *diverge* to maintain binocular fixation, even if my left eye is closed. The object of interest remains the "1" (because I follow Mariotte's instructions to the letter), but I see "0" with some part of right retina that's not the blind spot. Alternatively, in the vaunted moment of privation, if I move both eyes to bring "0" suddenly into view–closer to (or just on) the right fovea, because the left eye is shut–I've performed a rapid, *version* or *conjugate* movement of both eyes.

Specifically with respect to the latter (versional, quick) saccade, "[t]he visual stimulus for fast eye movement is target (object) displacement in space. . . . At discrete instants in time, control decisions are made based on the continuous inflow of visual information from the retina. In normals these decisions are essentially irrevocable; once the eyes are in motion their trajectory cannot be altered. The control signal is retinal error (disparity of image position from the fovea), which is automatically reduced to zero by the nature of negative feedback" (Dell'Osso and Daroff, 1978). Mariotte intends that I inhibit versional movement by "fixed and very steady" gaze on the "1," so as to keep "0" off the fovea and within the blind spot. If "0" returns to view with a saccade, I'm specifically accomplishing a reduction of disparity of image position from the fovea.

What, then, does cortex–any of the visual cortices–perceive during the experiment? And in the moment of privation, what does cortex momentarily *not* perceive, when a person observes that "0" has disappeared?

Aspects of what the retina "sees" reduplicate at every step in the entire visual pathway. The steps, in gross anatomical terms after the chiasm, include lateral geniculate nucleus and other structures that we might now entertain, including all the visual cortices from V1 to downstream, prestriate locales.

5

The Origin of Streams

For years in a building at the northwestern corner of my medical school's quadrangle, clinicians have taught neuroanatomy alongside neurobiologists. Shoulder rubbing, over time, has had a personal psychological effect: admonishment–in a nice way. Clinicians like me who simplify a subject to teach its practical aspects have a role to serve: we're on the quad specifically to keep "it" "real." But, compared to the scientists, what do I know? Fortunately, those people write, so I can read them in order to become, with chagrin over prior ignorance, *educated*.

*

All simplifications, even well intentioned ones, are hazardous when it comes to the nervous system.

*

Most of the fibers of the optic tract end in the lateral geniculate nucleus (LGN). So I have taught in class and on hospital rounds.

The purpose of this chapter and the next few (ending with chapter eight) is to discuss "streams" involved in visual processing. What is their origin? Our previous chapter clues us that the origin is retinal, not where the blind spot resides–though what the cortex perceives as a blind spot must have its origin, too.

The origin of streams isn't the LGN, the superior colliculus, or the **pulvinar** of thalamus. Most optic tract fibers synapse at LGN, but *some* optic tract fibers project directly to superior colliculus, bypassing LGN. In turn, superior colliculus projects to LGN and pulvinar. The latter projects to occipital lobe, as does LGN.[5]

*

In retina, axons that contribute to the optic nerve originate from **retinal ganglion cells**, whose cell bodies occupy an upper retinal layer, superficial to rods and cones. I consult a discussion of those ganglion cells in a colleague's review published in 2000–in 2000, I'd been teaching for about eight years; 20 years later, I write this monograph with that colleague echoing in my head with his redoubtable, Italian accent. Especially when discussing cortex in vision, we can't underestimate retina.[6]

Dating to the 1960's and 1970's, the article reads,

> [d]irectionally selective retinal ganglion cells were already known to exist, and improvements in electrophysiological technique have now begun to reveal additional transformations affecting the physiology of ganglion cells with simple receptive field properties. The retina works effectively across a brightness range of

---

5   One shouldn't conclude that projections to superior colliculus and superior colliculus to pulvinar are of equivalent significance to the termination of most optic tract fibers in LGN. I'm merely trying to describe a stream with rivulets.

6   He has written about retina–with its more than 50 cell types, many of whose functions remain obscure–as a "giant, incomplete jigsaw puzzle" (Raviola, 2002). I confess that, in thinking about the origin of cortical streams, i.e., retina, I assumed that the start of things must be simple compared to cortex. Such may not at all be the case.
    In this chapter, I mention neither koniocellular layers of LGN, nor the "W" retinal ganglion cells associated with them, for the sake of clarity.

10^8 intensity units, and this entails specializations at all stages of processing; for example, the retina adapts not only to *absolute brightness* but also to the level of local *contrast in the visual scene*. A striking recent finding concerns a predictive component in the responses of ganglion cells to *moving stimuli*; the cell somehow anticipates the arrival of a stimulus, increasing its firing before the stimulus reaches the region of the retina that would traditionally be defined as the center of that ganglion cell's receptive field [my emphasis] (Masland and Raviola, 2000).

Intensity units don't relate necessarily to color. Colored objects in our vision have a certain brightness, but color is both spectral and luminescent.[7] Adaptation to "level of contrast in the visual scene," however, has me think about the *color-related* problem of *constancy*, which we'll discuss in a moment. The excerpt also broaches neural response to *movement*, even the anticipation that movement will occur. Certainly, cortical processing has to do with direction, brightness, spectral wavelength, motion, prediction, among other aspects, but retinal ganglion cells are in much the same business, and they are physically closer to photons, rods, and cones.

Using our eyes as opposed to a camera with shutter and lens, "[a] white shirt . . . continues to look white in spite of large shifts in the spectral contact of the light source, as in going from overhead sun to setting sun, to tungsten light, or to fluorescent light. The same

---

[7] To illustrate brightness vs. color, Sacks (1993) describes his experience in testing the color blind: "I asked the achromatopes if they could judge the colors of various yarns, or at least match them one with another. The matching was clearly done on the basis of brightness and not color–thus yellow and pale blue might be grouped with white, or saturated reds and greens with black. I had also brought the Ishihara pseudoisochromatic test plates for ordinary partial colorblindness, which have numbers and figures formed by colored dots, distinguishable only by color (and not luminosity) from the dots surrounding them. Some of the Ishihara plates, paradoxically, cannot be seen by color-normals, but only by achromatopes–these have dots which are identical in hue, but vary slightly in luminance."

constancy holds for colored objects," writes Hubel (1995), who admired a Retinex (Retina-Cortex) theory advanced by Polaroid Corporation's Edwin Land. The simplest aspect of the theory is that, when it comes to vision, one can't discuss one (cortex) without the other (retina).

OK, so then . . . what?

*

Consider this LGN schematic:

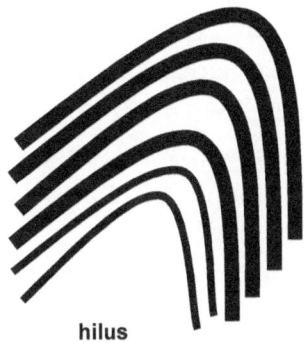

hilus

By convention, layers are numbered starting from the concave surface. The first two (rather thin) ones hug the hilus. The layers are thin, but they contain large cells, and are described as **magnocellular layers**.

The remaining thick layers, all dorsal to the two magnocellular layers in the schematic, contain small cells, and are termed **parvocellular layers**.

Due to incomplete decussation of fibers at the optic chiasm, a lateral geniculate nucleus in right brain (for example) receives input from both the ipsilateral (right) and contralateral (left) eyes. Textbooks teach that layers 1, 4, and 6 accept ipsilateral retinal input, and that layers 2, 3, and 5 accept contralateral retinal input. A point often not mentioned in basic neuroanatomy is that input isn't exclusively retinal. Indeed many other thalamic nuclei, with lateral geniculate nucleus as an archetype, also receive modulatory input from the very cortex or cortices to which a given thalamic nucleus projects. Even further, *other* structures, in brainstem or basal forebrain or elsewhere, also project to lateral geniculate nucleus (Sherman and Koch, 1998).

Getting back to input specifically from retina—sometimes called "driving" as opposed to modulatory input—we should be specific.

As in a recipe, fold in the following information (fair warning: the next two passages are taken slightly out of context; I'll justify my doing so in a moment):

> The visual system separates different types of information into parallel segregated streams of processing. In primates the tracts from the retina to the primary visual cortex (V1) are cleanly split into pathways that are relayed by the magnocellular (M) and parvocellular (P) subdivisions of the lateral geniculate nucleus (LGN) (Maunsell, 1992).

Then we add a weightier dollop:

> ... the different visual cortical pathways have their origins in two different types of retinal ganglion cells. One type (the P type) terminates in the P layers of the lateral geniculate nucleus (LGN) and has general characteristics which make it more suitable for *form and colour vision*, while the other (the M type) terminates in the M layers and has characteristics which make it more suitable for detecting *dynamic form and motion* [my italics] (Zeki, 1993d).

Neither Maunsell nor Zeki claims that streams result in mere "cortical prolongations" (Zeki's phrase) from retina to LGN into cortex.

Rather, the magnocellular/parvocellular division refers us to a distinction between

dynamic form and *motion* (magnocellular), on the one hand, and
form-color (parvocellular) on the other,

but, one wonders,

can those aspects of what we see really be separated?

We'll continue to trace streams, but we can anticipate an answer now: maybe we can't entirely vivisect vision. (Black, white, and shades of grey are colors, so what's color vision? We say that a static object with other objects behind it doesn't seem to move, but what does *that* mean, *not* to move? How do we know that the static object is in front, and others must be behind it?)

We need some help in organizing our thinking, perhaps in clarifying it as well.

Easily visualized anatomy (e.g., the two hilus-hugging layers of LGN as opposed to the parvocellular others) should guide us; if anatomy didn't help us understand brain function in a real way, why would we obsess about it quite to the degree that we do?

6

A Note on Geniculocalcarine and Corticogeniculate

In a rush to return to the topic of our first three chapters, finally, back to striate and extrastriate locales, it's easy to overlook a passing comment from a few paragraphs ago.

Most every neuroanatomy student has a notion about optic radiations (a geniculocalcarine tract) arising from LGN; about **Meyer's loop** (also described by Meynert, Flechsig, Probst, Archambault, and others [French, 1962]); and about a parietal radiation (sometimes called Baum's loop[8]). We can observe different homonymous quadrantanopias depending on lesion location, as is familiar to anyone who has endured some early medical-school quiz about visual-field correlations.

My discussion in this book focuses on cortices, so I'll defer discussing the optic radiations in detail, save for one big observation: Meyer's "loop" loops forward and around the temporal horn of lateral ventricle. It extends so far anteriorly that Meyer, writing in 1907, found it "peculiar" (Compston, 2005). There's been debate about the actual anterior extent of Meyer's loop *in vivo* in any given individual–a topic

---

8 I've made an honest effort to track down information on Baum, to no avail. Authors refer to two components of the parietal radiation (central bundle, dorsal bundle), so one wonders about the veracity of referring to a single parietal radiation in the first place (Rubino et al., 2005, Hofer et al., 2010).

of interest to those who need to resect temporal lobe in epilepsy surgery (e.g., Barton et al., 2005)–, but we won't discuss such nuances.

Instead, let's obsess about the idea that a sensory cortex projects back to a sensory nucleus of thalamus, presumably using at least some fibers of an optic radiation. Why would cortex do such a thing? That it provides "modulatory input" looks/sounds to me like the violent waving of hands, a *sotto voce* admission that we might not know why at all.

My curiosity can be rephrased: "sensory" connotes data INTO cortex (from LGN to V1); is that incorrect? Yes, it's correct, but . . .

*

Nauta (Nauta and Feirtag, 1986) runs a few numbers that we might consider:

> number of optic tract fibers that head to an LGN: ~1,000,000
> number of neurons in that LGN: ~1,000,000
> surface area of a primary visual cortex: ~1,500 square millimeters[9]
> number of neurons per square millimeter of primary visual cortex: ~300,000
> number of LGN fibers arriving per square millimeter of primary visual cortex: ~700
> number of axons projecting from a primary visual cortex to points outside V1, per square millimeter: ~200,000
> ratio of cortical output to input: ~200 to 1, conservatively.

The fact that cortical output, in part, directs back to LGN is curious enough, but in addition, using back-of-the-envelope calculations, sensory cortical output could exceed its input from LGN by two orders of magnitude.

Does a sensory cortex prefer to send rather than to receive?

---

9   In 1933, Filimonoff estimated differently; he thought the surface area Brodmann's areas 18 and 19 together was 7,800 mm², more than twice that of area 17; if he's correct, V1 would be about 3,900 mm² (cited in Horton and Hoyt, 1991). Later, in our chapter nine, we'll encounter a more contemporary number of 2,643 mm². Filimonoff's number decreases the quantity of LGN fibers arriving per square millimeter in V1, and increases the ratio of cortical output to input to roughly 800:1.

7

A Task

The job in this chapter is to make simple anatomic sense of a claim by Van Essen (1995; Fellman and Van Essen, 1991; Van Essen and Gallant, 1994). Based on study of macaque brains, he says, some 30 or so cortical visual areas have been identified. Over 300 connections among those areas have been described–the 300 represent about one third of the mathematically possible connections between the thirty-or-so areas.

Most connections are bidirectional.

There are 30-plus visual areas. That's the claim.

*

Let's list the areas.

The visual cortices begin with V1, as we know:

V1
V2
V3
ventral posterior
posterior intraparietal
V3A
medial dorsal parietal
medial intraparietal

parieto-occipital
middle temporal (MT)
V4 transitional
V4
dorsal prelunate
ventral occipitotemporal
ventral intraparietal
lateral intraparietal
medial superior temporal (dorsal)
medial superior temporal (lateral)
floor of superior temporal
posterior inferotemporal (dorsal)
posterior inferotemporal (ventral)
Brodmann 7a
frontal eye field
superior temporal polysensory (posterior)
central inferotemporal (dorsal)
central inferotemporal (ventral)
superior temporal polysensory (anterior)
anterior inferotemporal (dorsal)
anterior inferotemporal (ventral)
Brodmann 46
"TF" (per Bonin and Bailey)
"TH" (per Bonin and Bailey)

I don't indicate how areas in parahippocampal gyrus (TF and TH) link with entorhinal cortex and the hippocampal complex.

Van Essen says that not every area can be confidently identified and that not every area has clear or clean borders (Felleman and Van Essen, 1991). If we exclude those areas for which there are "significant" uncertainties regarding location, we generate a shorter list–as necessary, we check Van Essen's sources to attempt rough localization of the areas:

V1	occipital
V2	occipital
V3	**occipitoparietal**, Gattass et al., 1988
ventroposterior	**occipital**, near V2, Newsome et al., 1986
posterior intraparietal	**occipitoparietal**, part of V3, Colby et al., 1988
V3A	**occipitoparietal**, Gattass et al., 1988
V4	**temporo-occipital**, ventral to "V4 transitional," Desimone and Ungerleider, 1986
V4 transitional	**temporo-occipital**, dorsal to V4 but ventral to MT, Desimone and Ungerleider, 1986
parieto-occipital	**parieto-occipital**, Colby et al., 1988
MT	**parieto-occipital**, lateral bank and floor of caudal superior temporal sulcus, Desimone and Ungerleider, 1986
floor of superior temporal	**temporo-occipital**, caudal superior temporal sulcus Desimone and Ungerleider, 1986
medial superior temporal (dorsal)	**temporoparietal**, area of superior temporal sulcus, Komatsu and Wurtz, 1988
medial superior temporal (lateral)	**temporoparietal**, area of superior temporal sulcus, Komatsu and Wurtz, 1988
Brodmann 7a	**parietal**, precuneus
frontal eye field	**frontal**

To the degree possible if we look just at gross specimens of brain, it should interest us to know where the parieto-occipital and temporo-occipital borders are. The sylvian fissure, of course, separates frontal from temporal, just as the central sulcus divides frontal from parietal areas. Frontotemporal and frontoparietal boundaries don't factor much in our discussion. I'll speak my peace about the last of the boundaries, between temporal and parietal lobes, towards the end of the chapter.

*

The idea here is to simplify, so, to start, I'll consult lateral and inferior views of the macaque brain:

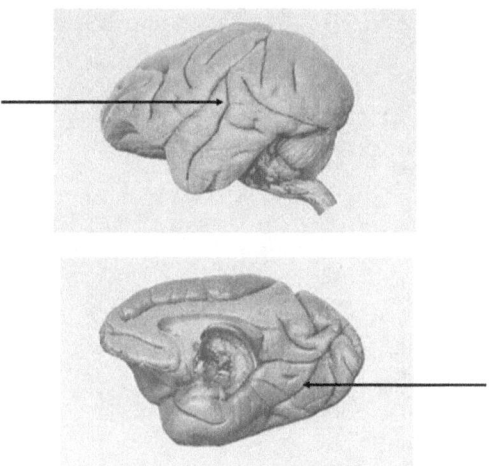

The top arrow points to superior temporal sulcus. The bottom arrow points to a sulcus that separates parahippocampal gyrus (medial to the sulcus) from everything else on the inferior surface of temporal lobe. I'd call it a homologue to the human **collateral sulcus**, which separates parahippocampal gyrus from the **occipitotemporal gyrus**, which is otherwise know as **fusiform gyrus**.

Keep this in the back of your mind (we'll come back to it later): superior temporal gyrus is in the vicinity of "middle temporal" or "area MT," also know as area V5.

Lateral to the single sulcus on the inferior surface, we visualize a temporal lobe area that extends into occipital lobe in humans, the occipitotemporal gyrus.

*

The parieto-occipital border is best visualized in sagittal midsection. The parieto-occipital sulcus, to be specific, separates occipital **cuneus**, posterior to the sulcus, from parietal **precuneus**, anterior to the sulcus. By convention, the inferior border of cuneus is above both the calcarine sulcus and the striate cortex.

Inferior to calcarine sulcus and the ventral portion of striate cortex is **lingual gyrus**, which can be tracked in more medial parasagittal sections into temporal lobe. The following image is Foville's; its unusual perspective allows one to visualize the extent of lingual gyrus towards mesial temporal lobe:

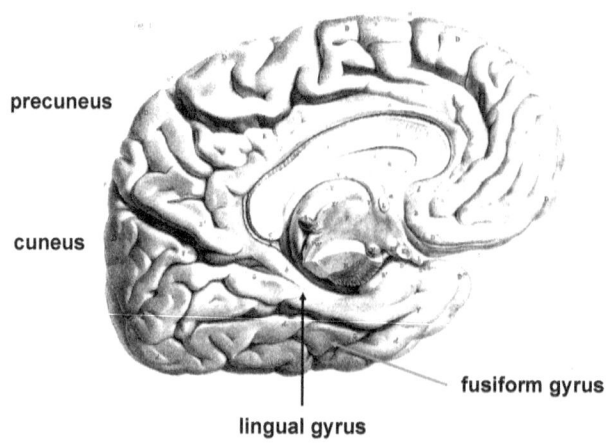

We've emphasized Meyer's loop's peculiarly anterior location in temporal lobe. When in the vicinity of Meyer's loop, we're near a *ventral* area V4 (Tootell and Hadjikhani, 2001).

Can we be more specific?

Sure we can be. Lateral to lingual gyrus is occipitotemporal or fusiform gyrus, which is V4's most probably location in humans (Zeki, 1993b).

Finally, let's gaze at a rather lissencephalic human brain at six months' gestational age (the cartoon is Broca's):

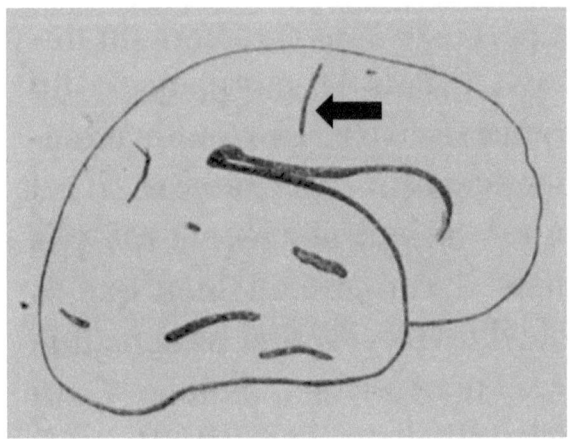

An arrow marks the central sulcus. Where's the boundary between temporal and parietal lobes? It must be at the very posterior extent of the sylvian fissure. Parietal, occipital, and temporal lobes converge where multimodal processing happens as a function of all three. Lobar distinctions blur in considering the cortical processing taking place at that confluence.

A metaphor from chapter two (Tootell et al., 1996) returns to mind, with a modification: if V1 were considered *just as part* of a bed sheet, then, in humans, that small part has been pulled around either occipital pole, and has been tucked into the depths of medial calcarine sulcus. The *remainder* (it's quite the extensive cover) *is* the cortical sheet that covers much territory in humans: both the medial and lateral surfaces of occipital and parietal lobes as well as the inferior surface of occipital lobe extending well anteriorly towards the temporal pole–in short, virtually all of the 30-odd areas reported by Van Essen.

8

Distinguishing Features of an Area

We've discussed Gennari's stripes, which we see on the ventral and dorsal banks of V1 on either side of the body of calcarine sulcus. A distinguishing feature of V1 is the presence of those stripes.

Also, V1 is intimately, physically proximate to the calcarine sulcus. If I miniaturize and position myself literally inside calcarine sulcus, with my feet one in front of the other at the bottom of the sulcus, I stand on the representation of the horizontal meridian in V1 at the bottom of calcarine sulcus. To either side of me, I touch V1; its cortical surfaces inside the sulcus face each other across my very narrow confine.

V2 is unique as the first cortical re-representation of the contralateral visual field after V1. Regarding medial cuneus dorsal to V1, we know about the V1-V2 boundary, defined by a representation of the vertical meridian, just above V1 (and below it as well in lingual gyrus, if we consider V1 below the calcarine sulcus).

From front to back both in dorsal and ventral V2, there's a kind of length-wise dividing line, not an actual sulcus, which depicts the horizontal meridian. The horizontal meridian forms the common boundary between V2 and V3–as distinguished from the common (vertical-meridian) boundary between V1 and V2. Then, at the superior border of V3, we again encounter a representation of the vertical meridian.

If we think clinically about V1 and medial cuneus and lingual gyrus, beware of caveats. First: posterior to the ventricular trigone in the subcortical white matter, there isn't a discrete separation of optic radiation fibers—actually, they jumble—prior to arrival at the dorsal or ventral banks of calcarine sulcus (Fraser et al., 2011). Second: there's a rule of thumb, useful to a clinician, that the further posterior a lesion is, the more likely the visual-field deficit will be the same in both eyes (a "rule of congruity"). But that's not to say that more anterior lesions can't result in congruous deficits, including homonymous inferior quadrantanopias which rather precisely respect vertical and horizontal meridians, associated with large middle cerebral artery infarction (Jacobson, 1997). Last: there are instances of cuneus lesions (tumors) *sparing V1*, associated with very clear homonymous inferior quadrantanopias (two cases reported by Horton and Hoyt, 1991). It doesn't surprise that the visual-field deficit in such cases should respect horizontals and verticals: both V2 and V3 are bounded/delimited/defined by meridians. But sparing of V1 is the curiosity. What information proceeds downstream, if V2 and V3 are damaged or even removed? What happens to information that presumably has already arrived at V1?

A 39 year-old woman (the first case in Horton and Hoyt, 1991) had a dense, congruous, inferior quandrantanopia that rigorously respected vertical and horizontal meridians, but she could perceive hand motion within her quadrantic defect.

Assuming that geniculostriate fibers aren't undercut in some way, shouldn't she *not* have a field deficit? And how is it that she perceives motion at all in the congruous quadrant of her blindness?

*

The thought that V1 should contain a complete visual or retinal database isn't a revelation, but, interestingly in the history of visual physiology, novel use of a stain helped begin to clarify the appearance of distinctive "modules" (of cortex; less a theoretical construct, more an architectural feature [Tootell et al., 1985])–modules which, taken together, process *all* retinal information:

> The scatter of the systematic topographic map of the visual field onto the cortex is such that, in the upper layers, one must traverse roughly 2 mm of cortex to get from one region of the visual field into an entirely new region. Any 2x2 mm block of cortex must therefore contain a complete set of whatever machinery is needed for the analysis of a particular region of visual field; it must take care of all orientations, both eyes and all colors, for, if certain values of these parameters are omitted, there is no other region of cortex to do the job. One can thus think of the striate cortex as consisting of a large number of repeating modules, all with similar connections and organization. . . . In 1978, studies of monkey striate cortex took a sudden spurt because of the discovery by Margaret Wong-Riley of a pattern of regularly repeating blob-like structures in the upper layers (II and III) of squirrel monkey striate cortex. The pattern was revealed by staining for cytochrome oxidase, a mitochondrial enzyme (Livingstone and Hubel, 1982).

In humans as well, superficial layers in V1 show "**blobs**" richly stained by cytochrome oxidase and, between the dark blobs, there are pale "**interblobs**."[10]

In contrast to V1, cytochrome-oxidase staining of V2 demonstrates modules arranged geometrically as **stripes**, not blobs:

> The metabolic architecture of V2 is very distinctive. It consists of a set of dark stripes running from the cortical

---

10 In the remainder of this monograph, I'll describe blobs and interblobs in V1 superficial layers, as originally discovered by Margaret Wong-Riley, although blobs may resemble columns that pass further into deeper layers.

surface to white matter, and separated from each other by lightly staining stripes. These stripes are not very obvious in horizontal sections but are well seen in sections which are parallel to the cortical surface. The dark stripes are then found to be of two kinds, thick and thin. Thus, if one were to survey area V2 in a direction parallel to the cortical surface, one would encounter cycles consisting of *thick stripe, interstripe, thin stripe, interstripe*, following which the cycle repeats itself [my emphasis] (Zeki, 1993a).

Unlike V1 and V2, V3 simply doesn't have a metabolic architecture, based on cytochrome oxidase staining.

*

Please indulge me: next comes a game of word association, a word-play made complicated by multiple levels. It's an exercise based on basic anatomy discussed since chapter five.

*

At a first level of association, if presented with the words

color and movement,

you'd think:

retinal ganglion cells.

*

At a second level of association, if presented with the words and letters

parvocellular (P) and magnocellular (M),

you'd think of both:

LGN and retinal ganglion cells.

Still at the second level of association, if presented with the words:

form and color,

you'd think of:

parvocellular, LGN, *color*, retinal ganglion cell.

Still at the second level of association, if presented with the words

dynamic form and motion,

you'd think of:

magnocellular, LGN, *movement*, retinal ganglion cell.

*

At a third level of association, if presented with

V1 blob,

you must pause, hard stop. Why? Because V1 blobs receive parvocellular and magnocellular input (Shipp, 1995 offers a very readable editorial on the subject). Magnocellular and parvocellular inputs don't segregate between individual V1 neurons or between V1 blobs and V1 interblobs (Nealey and Maunsell, 1994).

What, then, about . . .

V1 interblob?

Magnocellular and parvocellular inputs just don't segregate between blobs and interblobs (Nealy and Maunsell, 1994, again).

Keep in mind that the blob-interblob distinction is compelling by cytochrome-oxidase staining, and we may thank Margaret Wong-Riley for the discovery. But woe to the person who concludes that a "blob or interblob = either color or movement" in some mutually exclusive way.

*

At a fourth level, at very least (Sincich and Horton, 2002),

> V2 *inter*stripes

are associated with:

> V1 *inter*blobs.

*

Keeping things elementary, with the above information in your head, you can work backwards from a cortical area back to origination:

> area MT or V5/*remember*: in the vicinity of superior temporal sulcus on the lateral surface (parieto-occipital); V2 **thick** stripe[11]; V1 **(just "V1," because we won't obsess between blob and interblob in this stream)**; magnocellular; LGN; dynamic form and motion; *movement*; retinal ganglion cell.

Alternatively, you can work backwards from cortex in this stream:

> Ventral V4/*remember*: in the vicinity of Meyer's loop (temporo-occipital); V2 **thin** stripe; and V1 **blob**[12]; parvocellular; LGN; form and color; *color*; retinal ganglion cell.

One hears the screams of protest: so, what do V2 interstripes and V1 interblobs *do*; and, oh, why are we describing all this stuff in the first place?

---

11 Born and Bradley (2005), in a "gestalt map" ending in area MT, indicate that area MT's major input comes directly from V1, essentially bypassing V2, though they acknowledge a less trafficked connection via V2 thick stripes to area MT.

12 Sincich and Horton (2002) are explicit that V2 thin-stripe input comes mainly from cytochrome-oxidase rich areas of V1, especially in V1 superficial layers (2 and 3). If they're correct, a teacher's life is made a little easier: all V1 output (again, from superficial layers) is both parvo- and magnocellular; there are only two destinations in V2–on the one hand, thin stripes; on the other, both interstripes and thick stripes.

Interblobs and interstripes certainly must relate to processing beyond V2.[13]

That said, ...

... since interblobs probably receive both magnocellular and parvocellular input, a division between magnocellular and parvocellular streams probably isn't justified, not past V1.

*

Despite the known fact that all well-intentioned simplifications are hazardous, all this stuff is a form of play–some fun perhaps–, with basis in evidence.[14]

---

13 Based on functional MR rather than cytochrome-oxidase staining (Conway et al., 2007), macaque area V4 consists of "globs" (functional MR hotspots that seem tuned to color) and "interglobs." Don't let the nomenclature drive you nuts.
V4 globs (not blobs) are associated with V2 thin stripes. V4 interglobs are associated with both V1 interblobs and V2 interstripes. The main point seems to be that V1 blobs link eventually V4 color-tuned globs. A stream from V1 interblob to V2 interstripe to V4 interglob may relate more to form than color perception. *The elementary distinction in the text still holds: V1 blobs, V2 thin stripes, and area V4 together form one associative set; V1, V2 thick stripe, and area MT form a different set.*

14 In my summary of streams, I try to reconcile three depictions of connectivity (Van Essen and Gallant, 1994, Maunsell, 1992, and Sincich and Horton, 2002).

9

Omission Correction

Chapters five through eight have taken us from retina to cortex. We've simplified Van Essen's list from 30-plus areas down to five:

V1	occipital
V2	occipital
V3	occipitoparietal
V4	temporo-occipital
MT	parieto-occipital

By focusing our view, we'll benefit from much useful information about these five visual cortices in particular. In this monograph, other visual cortices find their way to the cutting-room floor, but not to worry: sometimes, omission helps understanding.

But I've not discussed columnar organization—it's a palpable mistake that I'll correct now.

*

In visual cortex, columns refer both to ocular dominance and orientation selectivity. There are right-eye and left-eye ocular dominance columns in a given V1, and if we examine just one ocular dominance column, we know that if you pass an electrode perpendicular to the cortical surface, neurons all along the orthogonal track will respond to specific orientations in the visual world (Hubel and Wiesel, 1977).

Then we found V1 blobs in its superficial cortical layers (II and III, above IV).

As you look at this next image, forgive the schematization: orientation columns should much thinner than dominance columns; the various orientation arrows are much more numerous than depicted, always at different angles of orientation:

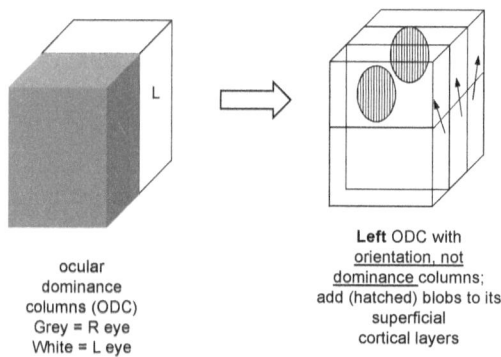

ocular dominance columns (ODC)
Grey = R eye
White = L eye

Left ODC with orientation, not dominance columns; add (hatched) blobs to its superficial cortical layers

One wonders what happens to ocular dominance and orientation selectivity as we pass from V1 to the four other cortical areas.

To start, let's peek at human brains with monocular visual loss (Adams et al., 2007):

> The occipital lobes were obtained after death from six adult subjects with monocular visual loss. . . . Mean V1 surface area was 2643 mm² (range, 1986 –3477 mm²). Ocular dominance columns [in V1] were present in all cases, having a mean width of 863 microm. . . . Human column patterns were highly variable, but in at least one person they resembled a scaled-up version of macaque columns. . . . In every subject, the blind spot of the contralateral eye was conspicuous as an oval region without ocular dominance columns.

Why select patients with monocular visual loss? The authors discuss one of their six cases in which blindness occurred at four months of age, presumably during a critical period for column "plasticity"; the associated V1 ocular dominance columns lost significant volume, but they *persisted* for a lifetime: "The most remarkable feature of this case is that the columns of the deprived eye survived, albeit shrunken, even after > 90 years of blindness."

Then, there's the issue of what happens in V2. The authors found cytochrome-oxidase stained stripes in V2, but couldn't distinguish thick from thin stripes. Based on experience in monkeys, early enucleation doesn't lead to loss of thick vs. thin, so the authors didn't think that monocular visual loss explained their finding–or, rather, their *not* finding thick and thin stripes, rather, just "stripes."

Nevertheless, by the time one reaches V2 in subjects with both eyes intact, architecture may have more to do with binocularity than ocular dominance, as a different research group has argued:

> In V1, where there are segregated left and right eye ocular dominance columns, the visual map is repeated, once for the left eye and once for the right eye. In V2, where there are three functional stripe types, the visual field is represented three times, once each for representation of color, form, and depth. This type of repeated representation results in an interdigitation of different feature maps. A complete visual field representation in one feature modality is achieved by a collection of discontinuous functional domains (e.g., a complete right eye visual field is achieved by coalescing all right eye ocular dominance columns in V1; a complete color visual field is achieved by coalescing all thin stripes in V2). Topographic representation within V4 is similar (Roe et al., 2012).

In V4, the same authors say, "Glob cells [recall information that I buried in a footnote from our chapter eight: V4 has 'globs' and 'interglobs'] are narrowly tuned for hue, tolerant to changes in luminance, and less orientation-selective than are interglob cells."

Regarding V3, it's been known for some years that its neurons are orientation selective (Felleman and Van Essen, 1987; Gegenfurtner et al., 1997); also, that those neurons may organize into columns despite the lack of a stain that helps in columnar visualization; and that V3 neurons also are tuned to disparities between two eyes in stereoscopic vision (Adams and Zeki, 2001). Of late, V3 columns selective for disparity have been identified in high-magnetic field functional imaging (Nasr et al., 2016).

I'm struck by the fact that representations of right and left eyes are clearly present in LGN and V1, but binocular processing based on an integrated cortical map of a hemifield may happen only as late as V2. Based on an amblyopia protocol in the macaque, unlike the human post-mortem study mentioned previously, we know that projections from V1 ocular dominance columns pass to binocular cells in V2; visual deprivation in one eye shrunk associated V1-dominance columns, but the effect *wasn't* "amplified further by attenuation of the amblyopic eye's projection from V1 to V2" (Sincich et al., 2012). What really happens at the interface of V1 and V2?

Beyond V1, a cortical area can map of a hemifield, with emphasis on central or foveal vision (area MT is classic in this regard [Born and Bradley, 2005]); an area can demonstrate columnar organization, but it may be tuned to visual aspects more-or-less specific to that area; beginning at V2, it seems that V1-dominance columns change their stripes, if the gruesome pun can be tolerated.

Writing some 40 years ago, Zeki referred to the areal representation *of function*: "a representation of distinct functions (in this instance, colour) with an arrangement of the cells appropriate to that function and not necessarily following any simple topographic relation to the 'visual field'. No doubt the representation of functions also determines the pattern of anatomical connections of these areas. It may therefore be more meaningful to ask for these and other visual areas, how a function is mapped, rather than how the 'visual field' is mapped"

(Zeki, 1980).[15] His comment is provocative mainly because one wonders where a visual percept (something identified in space) ends and where a "function" (e.g., identifying what it is) begins, as we'll discuss in chapter ten.

*

Let's end with questions and answers of the dreaded American National-Board variety, based on knowledge touched upon in this chapter:

Ocular dominance columns (ODC's) are specific to:

    A. LGN
    B. V1
    C. V2
    D. V1 and V2.

Answer: B. It's a bit of a trick question, since LGN has discrete representations of both eyes, but ODC's per se are associated with V1.

Word of caution: ocular dominance columns in humans are variable in dimension, not just because of antecedent monocular blindness, but perhaps as a result of genetic predispositions (Adams et al., 2007).

Next:

Orientation selectivity characterizes neural responses in:

    A. V1
    B. V1 and V2 only

---

15 There are reproducible aspects of an area's physiology—for example, neuronal receptive fields in V1 are smaller than in V2 and V3; in V4 and MT, the fields are larger than in V2 and V3 (Zeki, 1993c). Neurons in any of those areas (V1-MT) obviously respond to stimuli in an eye or hemifield, but there are differences in *what they respond to*, in keeping with enlarging receptive fields in different cortices. Areal representation "of a function" relates, in part, to what Zeki once admitted was his career "daydream" to demonstrate areas specific for this or that—color, motion, or what have you (Zeki, 1993c).

C. V1, V2, and V3 only
D. V1, V2, V3, V4, and MT.

Answer: D, but it's an unfair question, since we didn't allude specifically to orientation selectivity in MT. And only in passing did we mention inter "globs" in V4 and their orientation selectivity.

If, however, all five areas possess orientation-selective neurons, then what additional analysis happens beyond V1, especially in areas V4 and MT–the latter two having been linked to distinct streams and to putatively separate processes?

10

Why WHAT and WHERE?

What does it mean, to see? The plain man's answer (and Aristotle's too) would be, to know what is where by looking. —Marr, 1982

It's possible that the only sentence that I understand from Marr's 1982 book is the one used as the epigraph to this chapter—actually, it's his first sentence. I flip through *Vision* now and again; sometimes, I get ideas, whether or not they are Marr's in fact. Maybe the main problem I have with the book is its approach, which is called "computational." Since vision has to do with information and information has to be computed, there's justification, supposedly, to apply advanced mathematics in an understanding of how we see. If one isn't mathematically inclined, however, it's still possible to understand vision. There's only one indexed reference to "cortex" in Marr's book; he acknowledges that cortical areas exist, and isn't surprised that they might have different functions. That's all he has to say about the actual visual cortices. He's not into neuroanatomy.

We should spend a moment talking about the influence of one's approach.

Zeki has observed (more than once in his *A Vision of the Brain*, 1993) how the manner of your thinking can lead to anchoring bias. For example, if you visualize cortex the way Brodmann did, as a pastiche of so many areas with stained patterns of neurons in layers, then you might not be ready–ever–to ascertain anything beyond your stain. You're anchored to an idea *that a particular anatomy* reveals function. The approach, Zeki warns, may not be the right one to understand the subject at hand.

Much discussed in the visual neuroscience literature, there's also a problem in approaching vision as parallel processing. "The possibility that parallel streams originate in the retina and operate more-or-less independently up to the highest levels of visual cortex," writes Maunsell (1992), "has far-reaching implications for understanding the functional organization of the visual system and the nervous system in general." Read his paper carefully, and you'd sense that he isn't at ease with parallelism–or perhaps he's more comfortable with a thought that parallel lines can seem to meet at a distant horizon. Parallelism could be illusory. At best, it's just useful or heuristic.

So, what's wrong with utility?

> Although the number of cortical regions involved in vision is large, conceptually it has been useful to group both processes and their disorders into two main groups. A ventral pathway based on medial occipitotemporal structures appears to contain modules critical for object recognition and the basic processing of form and color that is required. A dorsal pathway based on lateral occipitoparietal structures is involved in motion processing and spatial processes such as attention and localization. Colloquially these have been dubbed the "what" and "where" pathways . . ..

That's Barton (2011). We learn from his article, as we'll discuss in chapter twelve, that clinical material–cases of occipitotemporal and occipitoparietal localization–certainly can corroborate a distinction between WHAT and WHERE. Speaking as a clinician, however, acquired syndromes of discrete cerebral dyschromatopsia (a ventral occipitotemporal disorder; think "WHAT") or of discrete cerebral akinetopsia (a dorsal occipitoparietal disorder; think "WHERE") are rare, frankly.

On the other hand, agnosias and aphasias, for example, are supremely common. Assessment of those two general categories of deficit often involve tasks that require visual processing, as when we ask someone to read a book aloud.

Like Maunsell and unlike Marr, we can trace streams anatomically. In fact, we *already* have, ending in our chapter eight. But anyone who even momentarily gazes at the maze that is "the hierarchy of visual areas" (the touchstone of all such images is probably Felleman and Van Essen, 1991, figure 4) realizes that there's *a lot of cross talk* in the hierarchy–a surfeit of railroad ties between parallel tracks. What's worse, the degree of side-to-side connection starts in earnest at the hierarchical level whose major players are areas V4 and MT.[16]

*

Among arguments to justify a difference between WHAT and WHERE, the best could be Margaret Livingstone's, in an unlikely place. Her *Vision and Art* (2014) comes from Abrams, a publisher of art books. If you're a museum-goer with a penchant for Impressionism–or, at least, an affection for Renoir's portrait of Madame Henriot (*look at the eyes*, Livingstone insists, on her p. 90)–then *Vision and Art* recommends itself for purchase.

For our purposes, read this:

> The Where system in humans and other primates is similar to the entire visual system of lower mammals. Lower mammals are less sensitive to color than we are, and they are not able to scrutinize objects and accurately discriminate them on the basis of visual attributes.

---

16 A vignette: in an impromptu talk on rounds, I once pulled up precisely figure 4 from Felleman and Van Essen, 1991. A medical student gazed at the image, and said explosively, "You've got to be kidding. This can't help me." Based on that experience, I specifically do not reproduce figure 4 from Felleman and Van Essen, 1991.

Instead, they are sensitive to motion, because things that move–either prey or predator–are likely to be important. Also, since the primitive mammalian visual system must have been used for navigating through a three-dimensional environment, it must have been able to process depth information and distinguish objects from the background. As the more complicated higher-resolution primate visual system evolved, the original system was maintained, probably because it was simpler to overlay color vision and object recognition onto the existing navigation system than it would have been to incorporate the two. The What system is a primate add-on (Livingstone, 2014a).

The issue is temporal priority–evolutionarily temporal, that is. *If* WHERE *is older than* WHAT, *then there's a reason to separate them, yes?*

*

Well, sort of.

For a moment, let's review. I've generally avoided reference to WHERE and WHAT prior to this chapter. But the reader knows about two streams, which we've traced from area MT backwards to retinal ganglion cell and from area V4, also in retrograde fashion:

> area MT or V5/*remember*: in the vicinity of superior temporal sulcus on the lateral surface (parieto-occipital); V2 ***thick*** stripe; V1 **(just "V1," because we won't obsess between blob and interblob in this stream)**; magnocellular; LGN; dynamic form and motion; *movement*; retinal ganglion cell;
> and
> ventral V4/*remember*: in the vicinity of Meyer's loop (temporo-occipital); V2 **thin** stripe; and V1 **blob**; parvocellular; LGN; form and color; *color*; retinal ganglion cell.

Livingstone says that the first stream (WHERE) is older than the second (WHAT), and that "the new What system needed to be back-compatible with the already existing achromatic Where system" (Livingstone, 2014b).

Let's say she's correct. What, then, about the unusual case of *Aotus*, a noctural primate who is color blind?

The large lens and rod-rich retina in the *Aotus* eye suit its nighttime-dominated life, but *Aotus* lacks adaptations found in other nocturnal mammals, such as a **tapetum** (a light-reflecting layer deep to retina). *Aotus* lacks photopigment selective for short wavelengths (think: blue), though it carries a gene homologous to the human gene for that photopigment (Jacobs, 1993; Jacobs et al., 1993). Biologists have wondered whether *Aotus* became nocturnal over evolution, and whether its ancestors were diurnal. Cytochrome oxidase study of *Aotus* cortex finds obvious blobs in its V1 and a complex staining pattern in its area MT (Tootell et al., 1985). Having identified inferotemporal projections from occipital lobe in *Aotus*, Weller and Kaas (1985) allude to a V4 homologue in *Aotus*. For this particular color-blind animal, evidence for a WHAT pathway may relate to its perception of form rather than color.

Or, is a WHAT pathway in *Aotus* a remnant attributable to some diurnal ancestor?

Or, couldn't we talk about a WHAT's WHERE system based on both form and location, with color added later?

Do you intuit a problem? There's "intermixing of receptive field characteristics in different streams" (Van Essen and Gallant, 1994).[17]

Livingstone doesn't flinch. Intermixing is fine and dandy; nevertheless, there are constraints:

---

17 The sentence is neurophysiology-speak. One can be simpler. In the 19th century, Helmholtz wondered about a relationship between perceiving the shape of an object and the movements of the eyes necessary for seeing it (Helmholtz, 1873, especially p. 304). If the eyes move, the object technically does as well (a movement of eyes relative to the object), even if the object is stationary in space. So, are we talking about form, motion, or overlapping form-motion? More recent investigations refer to Helmholtz's observations and to the larger issue of motion and three-dimensional object perception (Siegel and Andersen, 1988).

The second level of explanation for the segregation of our visual system is that it is more efficient to carry information about–and make calculations about–an object's appearance (its shape and color) separately from information about its position and trajectory. The different subdivisions can then be optimized for the different kinds of information processing they need to do. The brain needs to connect cells carrying the same kind of information in order to process this information, and it is more efficient to make connections between nearby cells than to wire together ones that are anatomically segregated (Livingstone, 2014a).

"Same kind of information" is a sticky phrase, because "same" *assumes* WHAT-information is all the same just as all WHERE-information is the same. All visual data encrypted in volleys of action potentials through one million fibers of optic nerve (information about color, form, motion altogether) are arguably all the same as well.

More specifically, Livingstone means that differences relate to viewing parameters: by analogy, in terms of visual acuity (say, "20/20"), we're more likely to notice small differences in the world if our acuity is higher ("20/10"), less likely if our acuity is lower ("20/100"). In humans, acuity–or "resolution"–for motion is lower than for color (~50% lower); but acuity for luminescence is ~2-3 times greater than for color (Livingstone, 2014b).[18] What makes for "sameness" is the respective spec-sheet, if you will, of the perceptual system in question, WHERE or WHAT. Her argument is faintly circular: WHERE differs from WHAT because WHERE and WHAT pathways have different specs.

Let me stop quibbling. I *buy* Livingstone's argument.

---

18 So: a little change in luminescence matters more–we notice it more–than a similar little change in color, especially in the case of blue colors, because blue cones are far less numerous (1%) than reds and greens together (99%). (As it were, we have far greater acuity for red and green, due to the human retinal spec-sheet.)

I only add a thought that isn't mine, but it obsesses me. In terms of proximity of relevant neurons, efficiency of their connection, economy of wiring, etc. isn't V1 itself a premier locale for *all* the necessary processing for vision? Here's a discussion of area MT (think: dynamic form and motion; WHERE) that I read very early in my preparation for this book; at the time, I barely absorbed the words, and certainly didn't consider the argument's relevance to other areas, such as V4:

> Overall, MT does not appear to detect or measure visual motion; this computation occurs in V1. It also does not elaborate substantially on this basic signal; for example, direction tuning is not much sharper in MT and speed tuning is not much broader. One of MT's main functions–that is, above and beyond what is done in V1–concerns integration and segmentation. Obviously, its large receptive fields combine information over space, and it integrates V1 inputs and combines them, at least under some conditions, to compute pattern motion. Its opponent[19] mechanisms probably have a noise-reducing effect (Born and Bradley, 2005).

The words bear emphasis: "*. . . this computation occurs in V1.*"

Maybe one could likewise argue that, overall, V4 doesn't appear to detect form and color, because *this computation occurs in V1*. In fact, *all* computations occur in V1, probably with the help of retina and subcortex. Above and beyond what happens in V1, maybe downstream locales in the WHAT pathway "integrate" larger receptive fields and "segment" what's interesting from the rest of crowded visual space.

---

19 The authors define motion opponency earlier in the paper. An MT neuron may preferentially respond to motion in one direction (A to B). If motion happens from A to B, but, at very the same time, the neuron is also presented with non-preferred motion (B to A), then its response is suppressed.

11

Two Problems with Diagrams

The first is: diagrams, once created, seem immediately incomplete, because they are. The second: perhaps they should be animated. I'd prefer to build my diagram in steps:

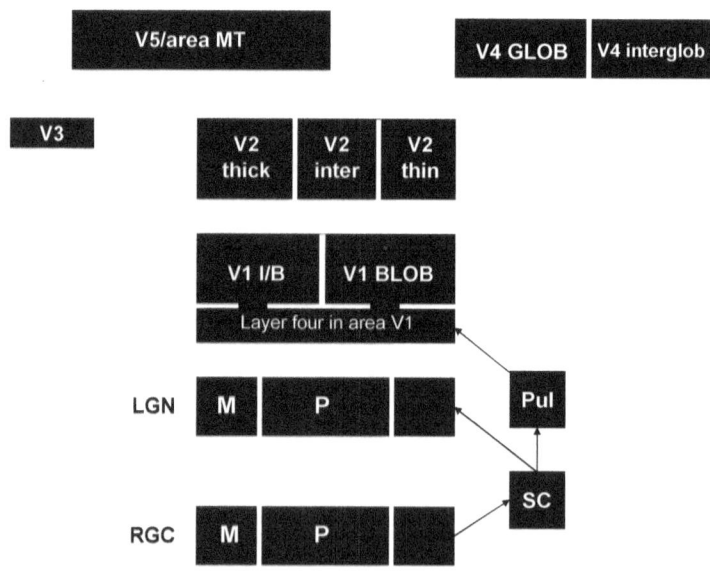

Black areas left unlabelled are locales or collections of cells that we didn't discuss. So, there's a population of retinal ganglion cells (RGC), neither "M" nor "P," that projects to SC (superior colliculus). SC, in turn, projects both to RGN to pulvinar (Pul). The latter, in turn, projects at least to V1's layer four (*recall Gennari's stripe?*). In fact, all projections to V1 go first to various divisions–even specific cell types–in V1's layer four/Gennari's stripe.

Other abbreviations are as follows: LGN = lateral geniculate nucleus; M LGN = magnocellular layers; P LGN = parvocellular layers; V1 I/B = V1 interblob + blob. V1 blobs and interblobs locate to superficial layers of V1 in my diagram (superficial to layer four). "Thick," "inter," and "thin" in V2 refer to differences in striped staining in V2.

*

Next, add links up to V1, but proceed no further than V1:

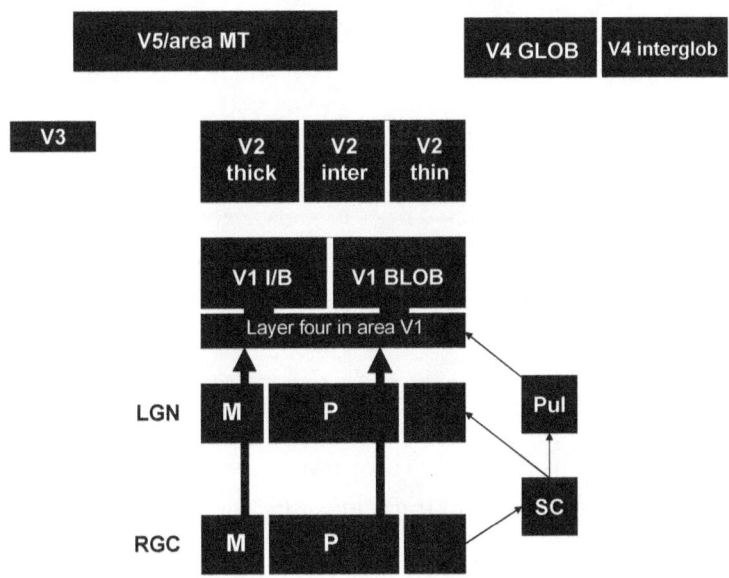

In deference to Livingstone's thought that WHERE is older, let's add relevant arrows for that stream:

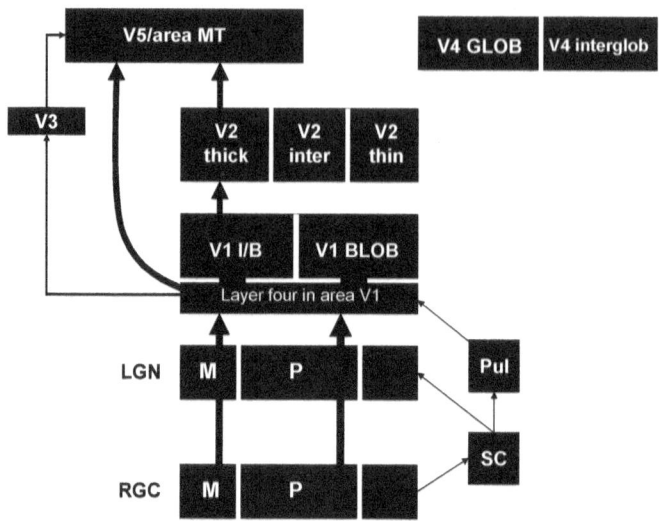

Born and Bradley (2005) say that there's a direct projection from V1 (from V1's layer four) to area MT, so I include it. They also think that a projection via V2 thick stripes is a relatively minor pathway, but I include it in the diagram as a robust connection, as discussed in our text.

V3 is of interest, because it doesn't have much to do with the WHAT stream, just with the WHERE.

Lastly, we incorporate aspects of the purportedly later system in evolution, related both to form and color. Although the discovery of globs and interglobs in area V4 is of recent vintage, I bring some (not all) connections to globs and interglobs into the scheme:

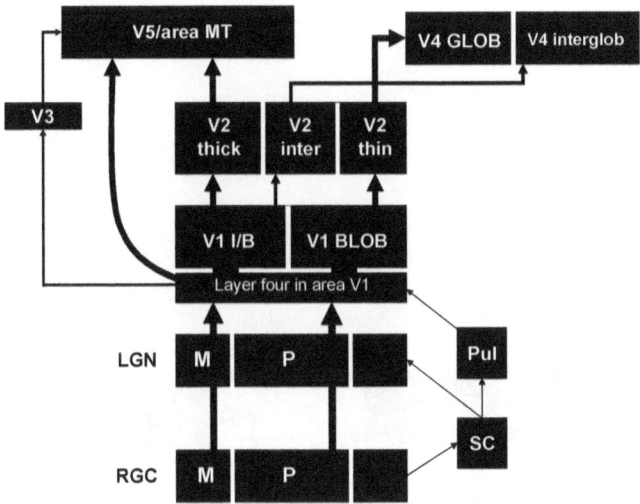

Thickness of arrows refers, very roughly, to strength of connections.

Question: why wouldn't there be a direct connection between V1 and V4? And don't V4 and V5/area MT connect? Answer: yes, on both counts (Felleman and Van Essen, 1991, figure 4).

And, naturally, there are other connections as well.

I'll stick with the simplifications of our chapter eight and will end with a un-fussy diagram to aid greater comprehension:

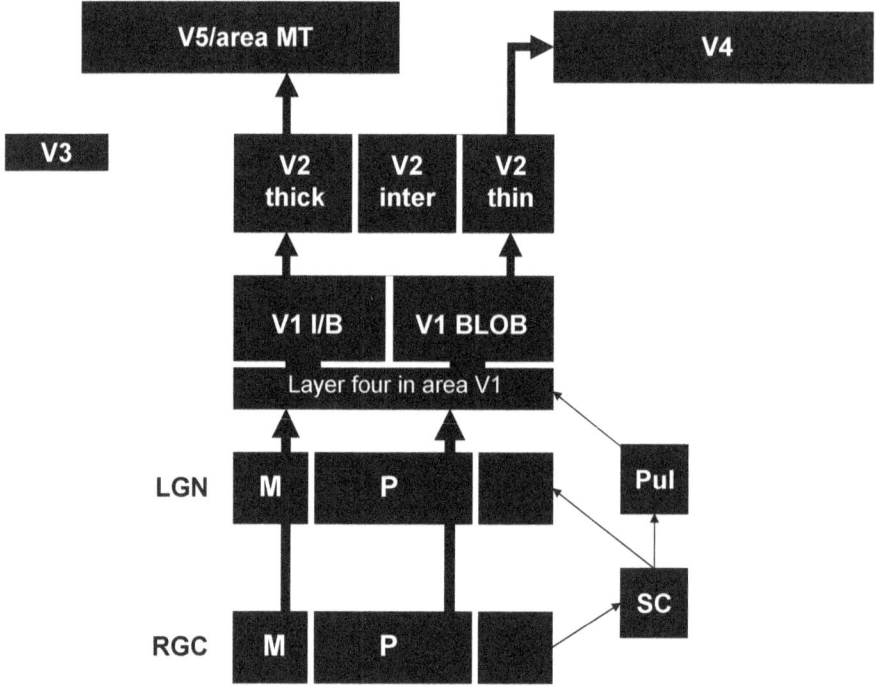

12

The Many Disorders of Higher Visual Processing

Concluding a short book, no one of right mind would encyclopedically take on the topic identified in this chapter's title.

We've described just one clinical case in our chapter eight; I had a question or two about her, especially regarding an ability to perceive something in a blind area. The story was: she had a dense, homonymous, inferior quandrantanopia, but she could perceive "gross hand motion" within her quadrantic defect (Horton and Hoyt, 1991).

How could she see that?[20]

Please don't rush to talk about how V1 could have a direct connection to V5 in the dorsal WHERE pathway. The whole point in discussing the visual cortices in the way that we have is to underscore that "higher" processing has much to do with lobar interfaces, particularly occipitotemporal and occipitoparietal.

In discussing those borderzones, the syndromes that come to mind are daunting, both in number and variety. Over time (decades), I've

---

20 The question has to do with **Riddoch's phenomenon**, which "involves perception of moving targets in a field otherwise blind to static stimuli from occipital lesions" (Biousse and Newman, 2009). The story about how George Riddoch was roundly chastised because of his observation, then ignored in the literature is told in Zeki, 1991.

patched together a way of thinking about many of them, of course with help (in particular, Farah's *Visual Agnosia* [1990]; for this chapter, I use Barton, 2011 as well several sources that I'll cite specifically in what follows).

*

At the bedside, when it comes to the array of disorders we're about to outline, an examiner develops an odd feeling (how vague of me!) that speaks to a question about what seeing *is* in the first place.

Consider a case from our service, discussed among us some time ago:[21] a patient was able to identify an orange (the fruit) presented to him; then he was asked what color the fruit was, and he couldn't respond correctly. He reiterated, "it's *an* orange." His visual acuity was fine and he had no visual field defect.

Was he anomic for orange?

Was he otherwise anomic or aphasic? (Answer: basically, no.)

Weird, right?

*

We can attempt a systematic approach.
1. First of all, let's introduce **agnosia**, a very general term used to describe the absence of knowledge about something. An anomia is an agnosia. So is an anosognosia or a simultanagnosia. There are many agnosias.
2. Types of **visual agnosia** include the **apperceptive** and the **associative**. For both types, visual acuity is OK; visual fields are (generally) OK; attentiveness is good enough to proceed with one's examination.
3. Example of an **apperceptive** agnosia, in what Farah (1990) calls a "narrow sense": you try to test acuity with a Snellen chart, but

---

21 I'm grateful to J.P. Klein of my hospital for his case description (initially, in a text message) and for our discussion about it.

Also, much of my clinical thinking about vision in general has been influenced by S. Prasad, also of my hospital.

the patient can't name letters. But she can indicate the direction of an E in the "tumbling E" test. Her problem isn't blindness or visual acuity. She does, however, have a problem with *the perception* of shapes.

4. We often ask a patient to copy a diagram (whether the intersecting pentagons of the Mini-Mental Status Examination or a more complex task). In copying images with details (for example, a house with windows or a front door), a problem depicting the overall gestalt of a house may speak to a **visuospatial apraxia** referable to non-dominant hemisphere, although poor reproduction of details–with comparatively preserved sense of gestalt–may relate to a dominant hemispheric component to the apraxia. The basis of the gestalt-versus-detail tenet goes back decades (e.g., Warrington et al., 1966). Yet thinking about point 3, all we need surmise that is the apraxia is apperceptive, in the absence of a problem with acuity or a visual field defect. Further power to localize has been debated (Guérin et al., 1999 and even in Warrington et al., 1966).

5. Example of an **associative** agnosia, again in a narrow sense (Lissauer in the 19th century spoke of a normal percept "stripped" of a meaning): present her a reflex hammer–just visually; don't hand it to her yet; she can't name it. Now let her take the hammer in her hand; she mimics hammering; after holding it in hand, she can name "hammer."

6. You could call the finding in point 5 an instance of "optic aphasia" (an inability to name an item presented only visually). **Optic aphasia** is a lateralizing sign, perhaps, referable to the dominant lobe. But associative agnosias often happen in bilateral hemispheric processes.

7. Example of **apperceptive agnosia** in a broader sense than point 3: **simultanagnosia**. We test it routinely using the "cookie-theft" picture, used, for example, in the NIH Stroke Scale. To state the obvious, there's *a lot going on* in the picture. An inability to narrate "what's going on" is simultanagnosic. There are at least two ways to fail the test.

8. Types of simultanagnosia: a. getting stuck on just one aspect of the picture; b. needing to identify the picture part by part. Either way, "what's going on" is hard to determine.

    In the first type of simultanagnosia, a person also demonstrates a hard time reading textual material; she basically can't. The second type can read a text, but she goes letter by letter slowly–sometimes, excruciatingly so. Both types of problems in simultanagnosia keep company with degrees of **alexia**.

9. I know that, in a reflexive way, simultanagnosia is associated with biooccipital lesions, as in **Bálint's syndrome**. A way to put the three components of Bálint's together is to think that the eyes get stuck **somewhere**. Therefore, she can't look at a new object in space on command **(optic apraxia)**; can't get a finger to a target presented to her in visual space **(optic apraxia)**, AND there's simultanagnosia, all as a consequence of the same problem. Thinking about that fundamental flaw common to all three aspects, one could refer to a **DORSAL/parieto-occipital simultanagnosia (apperceptive)**, because, if you'll allow use of WHERE language (in New England-ese, as a person from Maine might say), her eyes "can't get there from here."

10. Refer back to point 8. The second type of problem (the need to identify an image, text, or scene part by part, letter by letter, or object by object) refers to a **VENTRAL simultanagnosia**: "In ventral simultanagosia, *recognition* is piecemeal, that is, limited to one object at a time, although in contrast to dorsal simultanagosia, other objects are *seen*" (Farah, 1990). It's as if a form/WHAT pathway is easily overwhelmed.

11. Imagine the difficulties reading a detailed map or perhaps using various landmarks to find your way home (**topographagnosia**, getting lost in familiar surroundings, may be associated especially with non-dominant occipitotemporal lesions).

12. As an example of a percept *stripped of meaning* (Lissauer's still-germane concept of an associative agnosia), consider "maxim 47" in Devinsky, 1992:

These patients look in the mirror and don't recognize their own image. When patients with prosopagnosia look at a face, they can identify the nose, eyes, cheek and mouth, and can describe the whole as a face, but they cannot tell you whose face it is.

Although prosopagnosia is defined by this impairment in recognizing human faces, the defect affects visually triggered memory more generally, extending to other classes of visually related stimuli. Thus, there is not only a defect in visual identification of relatives and friends, but also in recognition of specific types of cars (e.g. Cadillac versus Volkswagen), birds (e.g. eagle versus owl), trees (e.g. pine versus oak) and so on.

Prosopagnosia is a **(ventral) associative agnosia**, although I have to put "ventral" in parentheses. Large lesions can be associated with parietal deficits. There's controversy about whether a non-dominant occipitotemporal lesion is enough to result in the syndrome; the typical association is with bilateral occipitotemporal processes.

The gist of Devinsky's maxim 47 stuns me in the same way that "disorientation to place, time, *and* person" disturbs me (can a person really be disoriented to self?). Failure to recognize one's face is a percept stripped of one's identity.

13. An example of a **dorsal associative agnosia: alexia without agraphia**, associated with dominant parieto-occipital lesions that also involve corpus callosum (on the dominant hemispheric side). It's an optic aphasia for books–a reader's "shattered" world.[22]
14. A paper from 1914, available in English translation (Langer and Levine, 2014), should interest us. It's astonishingly short,

---

[22] I think about a famous case, with its many dominant-hemispheric signs, including alexia. But Lyova Zasetsky could write *automatically* (Luria, 1987) and did so for 25 years after his war injury.

just a page or so. After acknowledging a similar phenomenon reported by Barat in 1912, Babinski describes two patients. The first, when asked to move her plegic left arm,

> ... remained immobile, keeping silent and behaving as if the question had been addressed to someone else.

Regarding the second patient,

> When she was asked to move the left arm, either she did not answer or she simply said, "Here, it's done."

Babinski opines:

> It is, I believe, permissible to create a neologism to designate this state and to call it anosognosia.
> I have also observed some hemiplegics who, without being unaware of the existence of their paralysis, seemed not to attach any importance to it, as if it were a matter of an insignificant discomfort. Such a state could be called anosodiaphoria (indifference or unconcern).

Anosognosia may not be a disorder of higher *visual* processing. On the other hand, not seeing one's plegic limb as one's own, as can also occur, would need to be considered a dorsal associative visual agnosia.

15. Are there cases of relatively isolated **dyschromatopsia/ achromatopsia**, an apperceptive agnosia? Sure, they're associated with superior homonymous quadrantopias, leaving the dyschromatopsia apparent only in the remaining, inferior-quadrantic visual field. The culpable lesion is in the area of Meyer's loop contralateral to the field deficit (Paulson et al., 1994). Patients often aren't aware of their "profound" ventral apperceptive agnosia.

How about isolated **cerebral akinetopsia**, a dorsal apperceptive agnosia? Sure, the classic report is Zihl et al., 1983.

How about isolated **color agnosia**, a ventral associative problem? Yup (Kinsbourne and Warrington, 1964). A question arises about our case of orange anomia: is there another fruit or vegetable whose name is its color? "Carrot" doesn't count.

We were able to find a case of a 34 year-old graduate student with a selective **agnosia for fruits and vegetables** (Hart et al., 1985) both when he was shown them or allowed to touch them. Other dorsal associative identification of vehicles, other foods, and animals was fine. He could categorize "fruit" or "vegetable" when fruit and vegetable names were read to him. A peach or an orange in front of him, however, left him befuddled.

*

The last four instances are rare birds of diagnosis–just curios, like Riddoch's phenomenon, that encourage us to glean even more about the relationship between cortical anatomy, perception, and the sometimes remarkably specific difficulty that people experience in seeing what's where.

References

Page 2
https://wellcomecollection.org/works/n8q3qrqy/items

Page 3
https://wellcomecollection.org/works/h4x5wjuh/items?canvas=115&sierraId=b2170935x&langCode=lat

Page 4
https://wellcomecollection.org/works/r6kzpkpr/items?canvas=837&sierraId=b28717752&langCode=fre

Page 29
https://www.biodiversitylibrary.org/item/131553#page/131/mode/1up

Page 30
https://wellcomecollection.org/works/ng6rx7bf/items

Page 31
https://wellcomecollection.org/works/r6kzpkpr/items?canvas=603&sierraId=b28717752&langCode=fre

All the above images are in the public domain. The author thanks The Wellcome Collection and The Biodiversity Heritage Library for the availability of their remarkable resources.

*

Books and Monographs

Biousse, Valérie and Newman, Nancy J. *Neuro-Ophthalmology Illustrated*. New York and Stuttgart: Thieme, 2009.

Brodmann, Korbinian. *Brodmann's Localisation in the Cerebral Cortex*. [Trans. and ed. Garey, L.J. from the 1909 edition in German] New York: Springer, 2006.

Devinsky, Orrin. *Behavioral Neurology. 100 Maxims*. St. Louis: Mosby Year Book, 1992.

Farah, Martha J. *Visual Agnosia. Disorders of Object Recognition and What They Tell Us about Normal Vision*. Cambridge and London: MIT Press, 1990.

Glaser, Joel S. [Ed.]. *Neuro-ophthalmology* [2nd ed.]. Philadelphia: Lippincott, 1990.

Helmholtz H. *Popular Lectures on Scientific Subjects*. [Ed. and Trans. Atkinson, E. from German] New York: D. Appleton, 1873. Available on line at https://doi.org/10.5962/bhl.title.29497.

Hubel, David H. *Eye, Brain, and Vision*. New York: Scientific American Library, 1995.

Livingstone, Margaret. *Vision and Art: The Biology of Seeing* [revised and expanded]. New York: Abrams, 2014.

Luria, A. R. *The Man with a Shattered World. The History of a Brain Wound*. [Trans. Solotaroff, L. from Russian] Cambridge: Harvard, 1987.

Marr, David. *Vision. A Computational Investigation into the Human Representation and Processing of Visual Information*. San Francisco: W.H. Freeman, 1982.

Nauta, Walle J. H. and Feirtag, Michael. *Fundamental Neuroanatomy*. New York: W. H. Freeman, 1986.

Nieuwenhuys, Rudolf, Voogd, Jan, and van Huijzen, Christiaan. *The Human Central Nervous System* [4th ed.]. Berlin, Heidelberg, New York: Springer-Verlag, 2008.

Sacks, Oliver. *The Island of the Colorblind*. New York: Vintage, 1998.

Shepherd, Gordon M. [Ed.]. *The Synaptic Organization of the Brain* [4th ed.]. New York: Oxford, 1998.

Talairach, Jean and Tournoux Pierre. *Co-Planar Stereotaxic Atlas of the Human Brain. 3-Dimensional Proportional System: An Approach to Cerebral Imaging.* [Trans. Rayport M. from French] Stuttgart and New York: Georg Thieme Verlag, 1988.

Zeki, Semir. *A Vision of the Brain.* Oxford: Blackwell Scientific Publications, 1993.

*

Articles and Specific Chapters in Books

Adams DL, Sincich LC, Horton JC. Complete pattern of ocular dominance columns in human primary visual cortex. *Journal of Neuroscience* 2007;27:10391-10403.

Adams DL and Zeki S. Functional organization of macaque V3 for stereoscopic depth. *Journal of Neurophysiology* 2001;86:2195-2203.

Allman JM and Kaas JH. A representation of the visual field in the caudal third of the middle temporal gyrus of the owl monkey (*Aotus trivirgatus*). *Brain Research* 1971;31:85-105

Allman JM and Kaas JH. A crescent-shaped cortical visual area surrounding the middle temporal area (MT) in the owl monkey (*Aotus trivirgatus*). *Brain Research* 1974:81:199-213.

Barton JJS. Disorders of higher visual processing. In: *Handbook of Clinical Neurology*, vol. 102 (3rd series), *Neuro-ophthalmology.* Eds. Kennard C and Leigh RL. Amsterdam: Elsevier, 2011, pp. 223-261.

Barton JJS, Hefter R, Chang B, Schomer D, Drislane F. The field defects of anterior temporal lobectomy: a quantitative reassessment of Meyer's loop. *Brain* 2005;128:2123-2133.

Born RT and Bradley DC. Structure and function of visual area MT. *Annual Review of Neuroscience* 2005;28:157-189.

Brodmann K. Variations in cortical architectonics. In: *Brodmann's Localisation in the Cerebral Cortex.* [trans. and ed. Garey, LJ from the 1909 edition in German] New York: Springer, 2006, pp. 181-201.

Choudhury BP, Whitteridge D, Wilson ME. The function of the callosal connections of the visual cortex. *Quarterly Journal of Experimental Physiology and Cognate Medical Sciences* 1965;50:214-219.

Clarke S and Miklossy J. Occipital cortex in man: organization of callosal connections, related myelo- and cytoarchitecture, and putative boundaries of functional visual areas. *Journal of Comparative Neurology* 1990;298:188-214.

Coggan DD, Allen LA, Farrar ORH, Gouws AD, Morland AB, Baker DH, Andrews TJ. Differences in selectivity to natural images in early visual areas (V1-V3). www.naturecom/scientific reports 2017, 7: 2444; doi:10.1038/s41598-017-02569-4.

Colby CL, Gattass R, Olson CR, Gross CG. Topographical organization of cortical afferents to extrastriate visual area PO in the macaque: a dual tracer study. *Journal of Comparative Neurology* 1988;269:392-413.

Compton A. From the archives. *Brain* 2005;128:1959-1961.

Conway BR, Moeller S, Tsao DY. Specialized color modules in macaque extrastriate cortex. *Neuron* 2007;56:560-573.

Dell'Osso LF and Daroff RB. Eye movement characteristics and recording techniques. In: *Neuro-ophthalmology* [2nd ed.]. Ed. Glaser JS. Philadelphia: Lippincott, 1990, pp. 279-297.

Desimone R and Ungerleider LG. Multiple visual areas in the caudal superior temporal sulcus of the macaque. *Journal of Comparative Neurology* 1986;248:164-189.

Eickhoff SB, Rottschy C, Kujovic M, Palomero-Gallagher N, Zilles K. Organizational principles of human visual cortex revealed by receptor mapping. *Cerebral Cortex* 2008;18:2637-2645.

Farah MJ. The apperceptive agnosias. In: *Visual Agnosia. Disorders of Object Recognition and What They Tell Us about Normal Vision.* Cambridge and London: MIT Press, 1990, pp. 7-33.

Felleman DJ and Van Essen DC. Receptive field properties of neurons in area V3 of macaque monkey extrastriate cortex. *Journal of Neurophysiology* 1987;57:889-920.

Felleman DJ and Van Essen DC. Distributed hierarchical processing in primate visual cortex. *Cerebral Cortex* 1991;1:1-47.

Fraser JA, Newman NJ, Biousse V. Disorders of the optic tract, radiation, and occipital lobe. In: *Neuro-ophthalmology, Handbook of Clinical Neurology* [vol. 102, 3rd series]. Eds. Kennard C and Leigh RJ. Amsterdam: Elsevier, 2011, pp. 205-221.

Gattass R, Sousa APB, Gross CG. Visuotopic organization and extent of V3 and V4 of the macaque. *Journal of Neuroscience* 1988;8:1831-1845.

Gegenfurtner KR, Kiper DC, Levitt JB. Functional properties of neurons in macaque area V3. *Journal of Neurophysiology* 1997;77:1906-1923.

Guérin F, Ska B, Belleville S. Cognitive processing of drawing abilities. *Brain and Cognition* 1999;40:464-478.

Hart J, Berndt RS, Caramazza A. Category-specific naming deficit following cerebral infarction. *Nature* 1985;316:439-440.

Helmholtz H. The recent progress of the theory of vision. [Trans. Pye-Smith from German] In: *Popular Lectures on Scientific Subjects.* [Ed. and Trans. Atkinson, E. from German] New York: D. Appleton, 1873, pp. 197-316.

Hofer S, Karaus A, Frahm J. Reconstruction and dissection of the entire human visual pathway using diffusion tensor MRI. *Frontiers in Neuroanatomy* 2010;doi: 10.3389/fnana.2010.00015.

Horton JC and Hoyt WF. Quadrantic visual field defects. *Brain* 1991;114:1703-1718.

Hubel DH. Color vision. In: *Eye, Brain, and Vision.* New York: Scientific American Library, 1995, pp. 159-189.

Hubel DH. The corpus callosum and stereopsis. In: *Eye, Brain, and Vision.* New York: Scientific American Library, 1995, pp. 137-157.

Hubel DH and Wiesel TN. Ferrier Lecture. Functional architecture of macaque monkey visual cortex. *Proceedings of the Royal Society of London, B* 1977;198:1-59.

Iaria G and Petrides M. Occipital sulci of the human brain: variability and probability maps. *Journal of Comparative Neurology* 2007;501:243-259.

Jacobs GH. The distribution and nature of colour vision among the mammals. *Biological Reviews* 1993;68:413-471.

Jacobs GH, Deegan II JF, Neitz J, Cognale MA. Photopigments and color vision in the nocturnal monkey, *Aotus*. *Vision Research* 1993;33:1773-1783.

Jacobson DM. The localizing value of a quadrantanopia. *Archives of Neurology* 1997;54:401-404.

Justel [Royal Librarian]. Mons. L'Abbe Mariotte's new discovery touching vision; with Mons. Pecquet's Answer [1668]. In: *Philosophical Transactions of the Royal Society from Their Commencement, in 1665, to the year 1800* [abridged], London: Baldwin, 1809, pp. 243-246. Available on line at http://hdl.handle.net/2027/mdp.39015073731393.

Kaas JH. Theories of visual cortex organization in primates: areas of the third level. In: *Progress in Brain Research*, vol. 112, Eds. Norita M, Bando T, and Stein B. Amsterdam: Elsevier, 1996, pp. 213-221.

Kinsbourne M and Warrington EK. Observations on colour agnosia. *Journal of Neurology, Neurosurgery, and Psychiatry* 1964:27:296-299.

Komatsu H and Wurtz RH. Relation of cortical areas MT and MST to pursuit eye movements. I. Localization and visual properties of neurons. *Journal of Neurophysiology* 1988;60:580-603.

Langer KG and Levine DN. Babinski J. (1914). Contribution to the study of the mental disorders in hemiplegia of organic cerebral origin (anosognosia) translated from the original *Contribution à l'étude des troubles mentaux dans l'hémiplégie organique cérébrale (anosognosie)*. Cortex;2014:61:5-8.

Livingstone M (2014a). Where vs. what. In: *Vision and Art: The Biology of Seeing* [revised and expanded]. New York: Abrams, 2014, pp. 118-127.

Livingstone M (2014b). Television, movies, and computer graphics. In: *Vision and Art: The Biology of Seeing* [revised and expanded]. New York: Abrams, 2014, pp. 210-219.

Livingstone MS and Hubel DH. Thalamic inputs to cytochrome oxidase-rich regions in monkey visual cortex. *Proceedings of the National Academy of Sciences, USA* 1982;79:6098-6101.

Masland RH and Raviola E. Confronting complexity: strategies for understanding the microcircuitry of the retina. *Annual Review of Neuroscience* 2000;23:269-284.

Maunsell JAR. Functional visual streams. *Current Opinion in Neurobiology* 1992;2:506-510.

Myers RE. Commissural connections between occipital lobes of the monkey. *Journal of Comparative Neurology* 1962;118:1-16.

Nasr S, Polimeni JR, Tootell RBH. Interdigitated color- and disparity-selective columns within human visual cortical areas V2 and V3. *Journal of Neuroscience* 2016;36:1841-1857.

Nassi JJ, Cepko CL, Born RT, Beler KT. Neuroanatomy goes viral! *Frontiers in Neuroanatomy* 2015;doi:10.3389/fnana.2015.00080.

Nauta WJH and Feirtag M. Prospects. In: *Fundamental Neuroanatomy*. New York: W.H. Freeman, 1986, pp. 308-315.

Nealey TA and Maunsell JAR. Magnocellular and parvocellular contributions to the responses of neurons in macaque striate cortex. *Journal of Neuroscience* 1994;14:2069-2079.

Newsome WT, Maunsell JAR, Van Essen DC. Ventral posterior visual areas of the macaque: visual topography and areal boundaries. *Journal of Comparative Neurology* 1986;252:139-153.

Nieuwenhuys R, Voogd J, van Huijzen C. Visual system. In: *The Human Central Nervous System* [4th ed.]. Berlin, Heidelberg, New York: Springer-Verlag, 2008, pp. 751-806.

Paulson HL, Galetta SL, Grossman M, Alavi A. Hemiachromatopsia of unilateral occipitotemporal infarcts. *American Journal of Ophthalmology* 1994;118;518-523.

Raviola E. A molecular approach to retinal neural networks. *Functional Neurology* 2002;17:115-119.

Roe AW, Chelazzi L, Conner CE, Conway BR, Fujita I, Gallant JL, Lu H, Vanduffer W. Toward a unified theory of visual area V4. *Neuron* 2012;74:12-29.

Rubino PA, Rhoton AL, Tong X, de Oliveira E. Three-dimensional relationships of the optic radiation. *Neurosurgery* 2005;57(ONS Suppl 3):ONS219-ONS227.

Sacks O. Pingelap. In: *The Island of the Colorblind*. New York: Vintage, 1998, pp. 28-57.

Sherman SM and Koch C. Thalamus. In: *The Synaptic Organization of the Brain* [4th ed.]. Ed. Shepherd GM. New York: Oxford, 1998, pp. 289-328.

Shipp S. The odd couple. Two distinct pathways in the visual cortex shadow each other from start to finish. Why? *Current Biology* 1995;5:116-119.

Siegel RM and Andersen RA. Perception of three-dimensional structure from motion in monkey and man. *Nature* 1988;331:259-261.

Sincich LC and Horton JC. Divided by cytochrome oxidase: a map of the projections from V1 to V2 in macaques. *Science* 2002;295:1734-1737.

Sincich LC, Jocson CM, Horton JC. Neuronal projections from V1 to V2 in amblyopia. *Journal of Neuroscience* 2012;32:2648-2656.

Tootell RBH, Hamilton SL, Silverman MS. Topography of cytochrome oxidase activity in owl monkey cortex. *Journal of Neuroscience* 1985;5:2786-2800.

Tootell RBH, Dale AM, Sereno MI, Malach R. New images from human visual cortex. *Trends in Neurosciences* 1996;19:481-489.

Tootell RBH and Hadjikhani N. Where is 'dorsal V4' in human visual cortex? Retinotopic, topographic, and functional evidence. *Cerebral Cortex* 2001;11:298-311.

Van Essen DB. Behind the optic nerve: an inside view of the primate visual system. *Transactions of the American Ophthalmological Society* 1995;93:123-133.

Van Essen DC and Gallant JL. Neural mechanisms of form and motion processing in the primate visual system. *Neuron* 1994;13:1-10.

Van Essen DC and Glasser MF. Parcellating cerebral cortex: how invasive animal studies inform non-invasive map-making in humans. *Neuron* 2018;99:640-663.

Warrington EK, James M, Kinsbourne M. Drawing disability in relation to laterality of cerebral lesion. *Brain* 1966;89:53-82.

Weller RE and Kaas JH. Cortical projections of the dorsolateral visual area in owl monkeys: the prestriate relay to inferior temporal cortex. *Journal of Comparative Neurology* 1985;234:35-59.

Zeki SM. Functional specialization in the visual cortex of the rhesus monkey. *Nature* 1978;274:423-428.

Zeki S. The representation of colours in the cerebral cortex. *Nature* 1980;284:412-418.

Zeki S. Cerebral akinetopsia (visual motion blindness). A review. *Brain* 1991;114:811-824.

Zeki S (1993a). The basic anatomy of the visual areas. In: *A Vision of the Brain*. Oxford: Blackwell Scientific Publications, 1993, pp. 94-114.

Zeki S (1993b). Functional specialization in human visual cortex. In: *A Vision of the Brain*. Oxford: Blackwell Scientific Publications, 1993, pp. 131-141.

Zeki S (1993c). The mapping of visual functions in the brain. In: *A Vision of the Brain*. Oxford: Blackwell Scientific Publications, 1993, pp. 147-164.

Zeki S (1993d). The P and M pathways and the 'what and where' doctrine. In: *A Vision of the Brain*. Oxford: Blackwell Scientific Publications, 1993, pp. 186-196.

Zihl J, Von Cramon D, Mai N. Selective disturbance of movement vision after bilateral brain damage. *Brain* 1983;106:313-340.

www.ingramcontent.com/pod-product-compliance
Lightning Source LLC
Chambersburg PA
CBHW021503210526

45463CB00002B/867